Comprehending the Nursing Process

a workbook approach

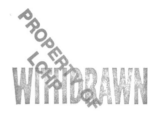
Comprehending the Nursing Process

a workbook approach

Carol Vestal Allen, MSA, BSN, RN

Nurse Educator
Veterans Administration Medical Center
Allen Park, Michigan

Formerly, Instructor
Division of Nursing
Mercy College of Detroit
Detroit, Michigan

APPLETON & LANGE
Norwalk. Connecticut/San Mateo. California

0-8385-7063-1

Copyright © 1991 by Appleton & Lange
A Publishing Division of Prentice Hall

91 92 93 94 95 / 10 9 8 7 6 5 4 3 2 1

Prentice Hall International (UK) Limited, *London*
Prentice Hall of Australia Pty. Limited, *Sydney*
Prentice Hall Canada, Inc., *Toronto*
Prentice Hall Hispanoamericana, S.A., *Mexico*
Prentice Hall of India Private Limited, *New Delhi*
Prentice Hall of Japan, Inc., *Tokyo*
Simon & Schuster Asia Pte. Ltd., *Singapore*
Editora Prentice Hall do Brasil Ltda., *Rio de Janeiro*
Prentice Hall, *Englewood Cliffs, New Jersey*

Library of Congress Cataloging-in-Publication Data
Allen, Carol Vestal.
    Comprehending the nursing process: a workbook approach / Carol
Vestal Allen.
      p. cm.
    ISBN 0-8385-7063-1
    1. Nursing—Case Studies.   1. Title.
    [DNLM: 1. Nursing Diagnosis—examination questions.   2. Nursing
Process—examination questions. WY 18 A4245c]
RT41.A43 1991
010.73'070—dc20
DNLM/DLC   90-14565
  for Library of Congress   CIP
Acquisitions Editor: Linda B. Nold
Designed and Produced by: Jolene Vezzetti, Mike Kelly, Janice Barsevich, and Steve Byrum

Reviewers

Marjorie Allen, BA
Graduate Student
American University
Washington, D.C.

Ann Becker, RN, MSN
Associate Professor
School of Nursing
St. Louis University
St. Louis, Missouri
Board of Directors
North American Nursing Diagnosis Association

Clinton Boyd, Jr, RN, MSN
Chief, Nursing Service
Department of Veterans Affairs Medical Center
Allen Park, Michigan

Katherine Johnson Bradley, RN, MSN
Associate Professor and Director,
Extended Campus
Division of Nursing
Mercy College of Detroit
Detroit, Michigan

Sharon Butler, MSN, RN
Medical College of Georgia
School of Nursing
Augusta, Georgia

Mary Deola, RN, MS
University of Michigan
School of Nursing
Ann Arbor, Michigan

E. M. Graham, RN, MEd
Lancaster County Area
Vocational-Technical School
School of Nursing
Willow Street, Pennsylvania

Joann Pieronek, RN, PhD
Associate Professor and Dean
Division of Nursing
Mercy College of Detroit
Detroit, Michigan

Susan J. Saydak, RN, MSN., CS
Associate Chief, Nursing Service for Education
Department of Veterans Affairs Medical Center
Allen Park, Michigan

Table of Contents

Foreword

The health care system is changing rapidly. Cost containment pressures are impacting on the length of inpatient stay. Clients receiving inpatient care are often critically ill. Complex health problems are still faced by clients discharged to their homes. At the same time, there is an ever increasing demand for health care services. The changing age structure in our society, is reflected in the increasing demand for such services by the elderly. The AIDS epidemic is demanding costly treatment. Improved and highly sophisticated technology is making is possible for segments of our society - such as premature infants - to receive such high tech care not possible previously. Then there is the push for health promotion and disease prevention: health care consumers today are seeking more information about health conducive life style changes.

The contemporary nurse is faced with caring for clients who expect quality nursing care and who expect the professional nurse as a health care provider to be well-informed. The contemporary nurse is also faced with caring for them following discharge in their home, while these clients are often still suffering from complex health problems. The contemporary nurse is best challenged with ever expanding opportunities in providing nursing care for a diverse group of persons in ever expanding practice settings, patterns, and organizations. The contemporary nurse is challenged to provide quality nursing care in an effective and cost efficient manner in this ever shifting environment.

Among the tools to help todays professional nurse to meet these challenges is the nursing process which can now be found incorporated into ANA Standards of Practice, state nurse practice acts, and major nursing textbooks in all specialty areas. This systematic approach to client care can facilitate the delivery of quality nursing care, and the clarification of nursing's unique contribution to health care delivery as well as the development of a common language for the profession.

Beginning students and clinicians need a means of clearly understanding and mastering the nursing process. *Comprehending the Nursing Process: A Workbook Approach*, is a unique learning tool designed for this purpose, examining the nursing process indepth in two comprehensive case studies. Part I includes an introduction, an explanation of how to use the workbook, and two comprehensive case studies. The first case study uses Marjory Gordon's Functional Health Patterns as the assessment framework, and the second case study uses Marilynn Doenges's and Mary Moorhouse's Diagnostic Divisions as the assessment framework. Part II includes clearly written explanations for each of the five steps in the nursing process. Interwoven in each step of the process are a variety of application exercises drawing on elements of the case studies to reinforce understanding. The exercises build upon each other to incorporate knowledge learned from each step of the process. By following the process, the user learns to write a thorough care plan based on the case studies in Part I. Part III includes a comprehensive appendix containing information needed to complete the exercises, and the correct answers.

The author - Carol V. Allen - brings to this project successful experience teaching the nursing process to basic nursing students and nursing staff. As a delegate on two People to People Nursing Delegations to the Far East and Eastern Europe, she has led panels and scientific exchanges on the nursing process, bringing much clarity to the understanding of this concept to our professional nursing counterparts. *Comprehending the Nursing Process: A Workbook Approach*, represents in written media much of Carol Allen's teachings from which many more nursing students and clinicians can benefit.

Gertrude K. McFarland, RN, DNSc, FAAN
Health Scientist Administrator
Nursing Research Study Section, Division of Research Grants
National Institutes of Health
U.S. Department of Health and Human Services
Bethesda, Maryland

Preface

Nursing faces two challenges in its efforts to deliver quality care in a rapidly changing health care system. First, today's nurses care for clients with more complex health problems than ever before. Second, nurses as individuals possess different personal traits and characteristics, as well as differing abilities and knowledge bases. The nursing process was developed to meet this challenge by providing nurses with a systematic approach to client care and a common professional language.

Comprehending the Nursing Process: A Workbook Approach is a learning tool designed to be used independently or in the classroom by nursing students and clinicians to understand and master the Nursing Process.

Part I includes an introduction, an explanation of how to use the workbook, and two comprehensive case studies. The first case study uses Marjory Gordon's "Functional Health Patterns" as the assessment framework, and the second case study uses Marilynn Doenges's and Mary Moorhouse's "Diagnostic Divisions" as the assessment framework.

Part II includes clearly written explanations for each of the five steps in the nursing process. Interwoven in each step of the process are a variety of application exercises drawing on elements of the studies to reinforce understanding. The exercises build upon each other to incorporate knowledge learned from each step of the process. By following the process, the user will learn to write a thorough care plan based on the case studies in Part I.

Part III includes a comprehensive appendix containing information needed to complete the exercises and the correct answers.

It is a pleasure to share with you the knowledge that I have acquired by implementing and teaching the nursing process. I welcome your comments and look forward to hearing from you.

Carol Vestal Allen

Acknowledgments

A special thank you to my children, Marjorie and Peter, my family, and colleagues for their continual support throughout this project.

I wish to acknowledge with gratitude the following people at Appleton & Lange who have contributed to the creation of this workbook: I would like to thank Linda Nold, senior nursing editor, for her constant support, inquisitive mind, and persistence in the pursuit of excellence. I would also like to thank Cyndie Smith, Jolene Vezzetti, Mike Kelly, Janice Barsevich, and Steve Byrum for their help in the production of the Workbook.

I thank Dr. Gertrude McFarland for writing a thought-provoking foreword.

I appreciate the valuable comments from Kristen Luke, a student nurse at Georgetown University, and her thorough examination of the workbook.

And through the years, it has been heartwarming to receive support and input from the nursing students at Mercy College of Detroit.

PART I: INTRODUCTION

THE CHALLENGES OF THE 1990s

The 1990s bring many challenges to the profession of nursing. In the healthcare arena, what essential role is performed by the nurse? Will nursing exist in the year 2000?

Establishing and identifying to the public the uniqueness of nursing remains a critical concern. A profession exists only as long as society considers the services rendered of value. Nursing needs to identify its contribution to the resolution of client problems.

The nursing process is the framework that enables nursing to identify its uniqueness to society. The nursing process facilitates identification of human responses to health problems. Human responses represent changes in the client's sense of well-being, wellness and life style.

The nursing process assists the client in achieving a maximal level of wellness, well-being and adaptation to life styles. The nursing process is operationalized through an assessment of each client and individually written nursing care plans. Nursing care plans customize the delivery of nursing care to clients and aid in problem resolution. The nursing process guarantees quality care.

It is essential to present the nursing process in a consistent manner throughout a program of nursing and a healthcare center. Consistency in teaching aids the student and practicing nurse in transferring learning from the classroom to the clinical setting.

The nursing process is (a) based on the problem solving approach, (b) founded on the American Nurses Association Standards of Practice (1973), (c) the basis for standards of nursing care and performance, (d) the legal framework for nursing practice, and (e) the core of quality assurance monitoring. Nursing diagnosis, step 2 of the nursing process, aids nursing in the transition to a professional model of nursing practice. Guidelines for utilization of the workbook, *Comprehending the Nursing Process: A Workbook Approach*, are discussed on p. 5.

PROBLEM SOLVING APPROACH

The nursing process is based on the problem solving approach. A problem is a question that is asking for a solution. Problem solving skills include the collection of information, the identification of a problem and the generation of alternative courses of action to solve the problem.

STANDARDS OF NURSING PRACTICE

Standards explicitly state the optimum levels of care against which actual performance is compared and measured. A standard of nursing practice focuses on the provider of the care, the nurse. A standard of nursing practice describes the nurses' methods in providing client care that assists the clients in achieving outcome criteria.

The American Nurses' Association Standards of Nursing Practice, 1973 (see inside front cover) define the role of the nurse in the delivery of nursing care to a client or group of clients. The eight ANA Standards of Nursing Practice state that nurses (1) assess the client, (2) formulate a nursing diagnosis based on the collected data, (3) (4) develop a plan of care, (5) (6) implement, and (7) (8) evaluate the effectiveness of the plan of care.

The American Nurses Associations Standards of Nursing Practice provide clients and nurses with written criteria for the evaluation of the nurses' role in the delivery of nursing care. Standards of Practice permit nursing to (a) defend its practices if the need arises; (b) conduct research to improve nursing practice, and (c) measure the nursing care provided to clients against the Standards of Practice for quality and appropriateness.

The nursing process is based on the American Nurses Associations' Standards of Nursing Practice. The eight standards are incorporated into the five step nursing process: (1) assessment, (2) nursing diagnosis, (3) planning, (4) implementation and (5) evaluation.

Professional specialty nursing organizations establish and publish professional practice standards based on the nursing process to guide the membership. For example, the American Association of Critical Care Nurses Standards of Practice includes the nursing process as a standard.

STANDARDS OF NURSING CARE

A standard of nursing care focuses on the recipient of care, the client. A standard of care states the outcome criteria and the care a client will receive from nursing service. Standards of care are established by nurses and explicitly state the nursing interventions that will be delivered to the clients based on an identified problem and expected outcomes. Achievement of the standards of care are reflected in the nursing care plans and nurses' notes.

STANDARDS OF NURSING PERFORMANCE

Standards of nursing performance compare the nurses' performance with the identified standards of performance specified in the job description for evaluation purposes. Annual evaluations of nursing performance reflect the nurse's ability to implement the nursing process.

LEGAL ASPECTS OF THE NURSING PROCESS

Malpractice stems from professional negligence. In order for the plaintiff, the client, family or significant other, to receive compensation for damages, the plaintiff establishes the following elements: (a) the existence of the nurse's duty to the plaintiff, based upon the existence of the nurse-client relationship; (b) the applicable standard of nursing care and the nurse's violation of this standard; (c) a compensable injury, that the injured client is entitled to receive payment for damages; and, (d) a causal connection between the violation of the standard of care and the harm the client claimed (Black, 1990).

Nurses are legally bound to follow the American Nurses Association Standards of Nursing Practice and the standards of care applicable to their work area. In a malpractice suit against a nurse, the plaintiff's attorney will examine whether the nurse, the defendant in the malpractice suit, implemented professional standards of nursing practice and standards of care. That is, the standards that a reasonable and prudent nurse would be expected to follow.

IMPACT OF THE NURSING PROCESS ON THE JOINT COMMISSION OF ACCREDITATION OF HEALTHCARE ORGANIZATIONS' STANDARDS

The Joint Commission of Accreditation of Healthcare Organizations (JCAHO) is an independent accrediting body. JCAHO reviews the extent to which healthcare organizations (e.g., hospitals) meet written quality assurance standards. JCAHO requires coordination of quality assurance efforts throughout a healthcare organization and involves administrative staff, nurses, medical staff, pharmacists and other professional groups.

JCAHO holds nurses responsible for implementing the American Nurses' Association Standards of Nursing Practice, and standards of care. The JCAHO Nursing Service Standards state nursing care will be provided to clients through the use of the nursing process. Nursing care is based on a documented assessment and reassessment of the client's needs (JCAHO, 1991).

IMPACT OF THE NURSING PROCESS ON QUALITY ASSURANCE

Quality assurance (QA) is the evaluation of nursing care against a standard. QA is an ongoing systematic monitoring and evaluation of the quality of care delivered to the client, the appropriateness of client care, the identification of opportunities to improve client care, and the resolution of identified problems (JCAHO, 1991).

Nursing service constructs QA monitors founded on the nursing process and tracts implementation of the five step nursing process. The QA monitor begins with an audit of the admission data assessment tool (step 1), the nursing care plan (step 2 and 3) and the nurses notes (step 4 and step 5). The QA monitor quantitatively measures the compliance rate with established standards of practice and care.

Quality assurance monitoring is usually conducted on a quarterly basis during a fiscal year. An acceptable compliance rate is established by the nursing service quality assurance committee. For example, in a hospital 91-100% of the clients on a nursing unit must have a written nursing care plan and documentation of nursing actions. Sharing results of the QA monitors assists the nurses in identifying strengths and areas needing improvement in their delivery of nursing care.

Student nurses and practicing professionals contribute to the quality of client care. The nursing QA monitors provide evidence to JCAHO and other accrediting organizations that quality care has been rendered to the clients.

FUNCTIONING WITHIN A NURSING MODEL IN NURSING PRACTICE

The uniqueness of nursing is readily identified through the application of a nursing model. When the nurse functions within a nursing model, the problems identified, the data collected and the nursing diagnoses formulated are different from those of physicians. Nursing models deal with human responses to a problem that fall within the realm of nursing care.

In a medical model, the medical diagnosis addresses pathological cellular, tissue and organ changes. Changes are identified through an assessment of body systems. For example, a physician will conduct a health assessment of body systems such as the cardiovascular, neurological, urological and gastrointestinal systems.

There are various methods to collect and cluster client data. *Comprehending the Nursing Process: A Workbook Approach* presents the assessment of clients using two nursing models: (1) Gordon's 11 Functional Health Patterns (Appendix A, p. 133-136), and (2) Doenges and Moorhouse's Diagnostic Divisions (Appendix B, p. 137-139). Functional health patterns and diagnostic divisions organize the assessment data according to human responses to a problem. Both models have been tested in nursing practice for several years. In addition to facilitating the assessment of the client, the models aid in the identification of appropriate nursing diagnoses, and guide the nursing plan of care.

BACKGROUND AND RATIONALE FOR NURSING DIAGNOSIS

Nursing diagnosis aids in the transition to a professional model of nursing practice. In 1973, the North American Nursing Diagnosis Association (NANDA) held its first conference. At the time, nursing lacked autonomy that characterized it as a profession. Nursing leaders strove to clarify the nurse's role in the delivery of healthcare. Nursing diagnosis was accepted as the term used to describe problems identified in nursing practice and within the realm of nursing to care. Nursing diagnosis became step 2 of the nursing process.

With an increase in the number of nursing diagnoses, a need to organize them into an orderly structure evolved. Consequently, NANDA developed a taxonomy to classify nursing diagnoses.

Nine human response patterns provide the classification schema. Nursing diagnoses are listed under the human response patterns according to the pattern definition, and the diagnosis definition and defining characteristics.

Each nursing diagnostic label in the NANDA taxonomy is defined. The diagnostic labels and definitions facilitate consistency, communication and utilization of the NANDA taxonomy around the world. NANDAs Nursing Diagnosis Taxonomy I was accepted by the 1986 General Assembly of NANDA. Taxonomy I-Revised (Appendix C, p. 141-142) was accepted at the 1990 NANDA Ninth Conference. The taxonomy has been prepared for possible inclusion in the World Health Organization's International Classification of Diseases (ICD).

Professional nursing organizations promote the formulation of nursing diagnoses. The American Nurses Association (ANA) supports nursing diagnoses. The ANA Standards of Practice (1973), Standard II states, "Nursing diagnoses are derived from health status data." The ANA Social Policy statement indicates, "Nursing is the diagnosis and treatment of human responses to actual or potential health problems" (ANA, 1980, p. 9). The ANA acknowledged NANDA as the association to be utilized by the ANA practice councils for the development, review and approval of nursing diagnoses (ANA, 1988). Nursing diagnoses facilitate reimbursement for nursing interventions.

NANDA remains the professional nursing organization responsible for the research, classification and approval of nursing diagnoses for use by nurses throughout the world. Every two years NANDA reviews and approves nursing diagnoses that have been researched and tested clinically for their inclusion in the NANDA list of approved diagnostic labels.

The Nine Human Response Patterns of the NANDA Taxonomy

Patterns	Definitions	Patterns	Definitions
1. Exchanging	Mutual giving and receiving	6. Moving	Activity
2. Communicating	Sending messages	7. Perceiving	Reception of Information
3. Relating	Establishing bonds	8. Knowing	Meaning associated with information
4. Valuing	Assigning of relative worth	9. Feeling	Subjective awareness of information
5. Choosing	Selection of Alternatives		

How to Use the Workbook

Each step of the nursing process is succinctly explained in the workbook and followed by an exercise based on either case study #1 or case study #2. The inclusion of exercises assist the user in (a) active involvement in the application of the five step nursing process and (b) the development of beginning critical thinking. The user, at times, will need to refer to information in Appendix A-L, p. 133-174, for information to answer some of the exercises. The recommended answers to the exercises are located in Appendix M (p. 175-209). The workbook offers the user an opportunity to select one or both of the case studies for each content area.

The case studies focus on a client's responses to a medical problem, case study #1, and a surgical problem, case study #2. The case studies are presented using assessment frameworks of nursing models. Gordon's 11 Functional Health Patterns, the nursing model used in case study #1, represent sequences of behavior that is, ways of living (Gordon, 1989). See Appendix A, p. 133-136, for Gordon's assessment framework. Doenges and Moorhouse's 13 Diagnostic Divisions , the nursing model used in case study #2, "reflect a blend of Maslow's Hierarchy of Needs and a self-care philosophy" (Doenges & Moorhouse, 1989). See Appendix B, p. 137-139, for Doenges and Moorhouse's framework.

In the workbook, the word client refers to the individual, family, significant other or the community. Outcome criteria are synonymous with client goals and objectives, expected outcomes, outcome behaviors, long and short term goals.

The author based the workbook on information gleaned from years of research and teaching of the nursing process to student nurses, registered nurses and licensed practical nurses. *Comprehending the Nursing Process: A Workbook Approach* focuses on application of the five step nursing process.

Case Studies

Medical p. 7-12	Surgical p. 13-19
Case Study #1: Human Response to a Medical Problem (Rheumatoid Arthritis)	Case Study #2: Human Response to a Surgical Problem (Carcinoma Left Breast, Stage I)

Case Study #1: Human Response to a Medical Problem (Rheumatoid Arthritis)

DEMOGRAPHIC DATA

Date of interview: 9/3/91
Client: Mr. James Hill
Address: 525 Westlady, Detroit, MI 48236
Telephone: 971-6288
Contact: Wife
Address of contact: Same as client
Age: 64   Sex: Male   Race: Black
Educational background: High school
Religion: Baptist   Marital status: Married
Usual occupation: Photographer
Source of income: Self-employed
Insurance: Blue Cross/Blue Shield
Source of history: Client
Reliability of historian (1-4): 4

ASSESSMENT OF GORDON'S 11 FUNCTIONAL HEALTH PATTERNS

1. Nursing History for Health Perception-Health Management Pattern

"This is the worst attack of arthritis that I have had in the past 30 years. For the past two weeks, I have had pain, swelling and redness of my knuckles, and they feel warmer than usual. I have felt chills for the past two weeks. All of these problems started three months ago. I had an infected bunion on my left foot. The doctor lanced the bunion and pus poured out. The doctor put me on antibiotics. When I saw the doctor 8/18/91, I could not smell or taste, and my mouth was full of sores."

Health record indicated that the client experienced an exacerbation of his rheumatoid arthritis signs and symptoms 8/18/91, and received a cortisone injection into his left wrist without relief of symptoms. On 8/18/91, the bunion was drained with the return of a copious amount of purulent drainage. On 9/1/91, fluid was cultured from the client's painful left wrist. The health record revealed that on 8/12/91 methotrexate 2.5 mg orally was ordered for 5 days. On 8/18/91, the client was diagnosed with methotrexate toxicity, and the methotrexate was discontinued.

<u>General Survey:</u> Sitting down on bed staring at floor during interview. Facial muscles taut. Holding sides of the bed for support. Warmth, redness, swelling right first and second metacarpal phalange joints and left bunion. Facial grimacing and moaning upon movement of joints. Lesions throughout oral cavity. Temperature 101 F (R). Diaphoretic. Ulcer left foot crusty yellowish rim.

Past Health History:	30 year history of rheumatoid arthritis; usually experiences three exacerbations every year. May take days to weeks to obtain pain relief with ecotrin. Treated with antimalarials and gold in the past.
General Health:	Rheumatoid arthritis major health problem. Denies shortness of breath (SOB). Decreased appetite and weight loss past month.
Prophylactic Medical/Dental:	Physical examination by physician every year. Annual dental visits.
Surgical Procedures:	Tonsillectomy 1940; implants secondary removal of cataracts 1986.
Childhood Illness:	Measles, whooping cough.
Immunizations Completed:	All childhood immunizations. Last tetanus 1985.
Current Medications:	
Prescription-	Voltarin 50 mg Tabs 1 (o) tid Tylenol #3 Tabs 3-4 (o) qd 9/3/91 Nafcillin 2g IVPB q 4h started in emergency room. Heplock in right forearm.
Nonprescription-	Ecotrin 325 mg Tabs 2 four times a day for past 20 years.
Allergies:	Methotrexate; grass.
Habits:	46 year history of smoking one pack of cigarettes per day.
Family Health History:	Maternal grandmother died diabetes mellitus at age 56. Father died cancer of gallbladder age 76. Mother died Alzheimers age 74. Cause of death of other grandparents unknown.
Social History:	Photography business in client's home. Married to wife past 40 years. Wife 60 years old. Works as a secretary. Five living children ages 37, 35, 30, 29, 27. Denies use of recreational drugs. Church functions comprise social activities.
Laboratory Findings:	9/1/91 Fluid from left foot bunion positive for staphylococcus aureus. White blood cells (WBCs) 11,000 uL (mm3).

2. Nursing History for Nutritional-Metabolic Pattern

Client states, "I prepare my breakfast and lunch, and my wife fixes dinner. I do not have food allergies. Now, I only eat a little food since nothing smells or tastes good, and my mouth is sore. I was allergic to methotrexate. I cannot chew with all these sores so I puree all my food now. I rinse my mouth with salt water after each meal. I have lost weight this past month. I eat balanced meals. My wife makes sure there is food in the house. I have given up using salt. We cook with vegetable oil and use margarine. I feel chilly. I sweat a lot. I drink 2 juice glasses of water a day. I do not eat between meals or snack.

Presently, Mr. Smith eats pureed food. Social worker's note in the health record indicated that client had a food processor at home and pureed own food. Physician ordered low sodium (2g), pureed diet. Ate 50% pureed lunch that consisted of peas, meat, fruit and skim milk. Twenty-four hour fluid intake 1680cc and urine output 1500cc.

<u>Typical Daily Intake</u>
<u>Before Mouth Lesions</u>:

Breakfast-	1 juice glass of orange juice, 1 cup of coffee, bowl of oatmeal with 1/4c. skim milk. One egg twice a week.
Lunch-	Tuna fish or ham sandwich on wheat toast, bowl of vegetable soup, fruit, 1 cup of coffee.
Dinner-	Fish, rice, green vegetable, toss salad with oil and vinegar dressing, 1 scoop of sherbet, 1 cup decaffeinated coffee.
Evening Snacks-	None

<u>Physical Examination</u>:   Height: 5'11" Large frame. Actual weight: 154 lbs. Usual weight: 165. Lost 10 pounds in past 6 months. Temperature 101 F (R). Skin hot to touch. Skin turgor: shape returned in 15 seconds. Diaphoretic. Positive subcutaneous nodules, firm on extremity surface. Hair sparse. No clubbing of fingers. Ulcers throughout buccal mucosa. Tongue and gums erythematous (red). Upper dentures; partial lower removed due to presence lesions. Lips, tonsils, pharynx, speech within normal limits (WNL). Increased oral secretions. Halitosis present.

<u>Laboratory Findings</u>:   9/3/91

Blood-

Serum albumin: 3.5 g/dL
Serum potassium (K+): 4.7 mEq/L
Serum sodium (Na+): 133 mEq/L
Glucose: 105 mg/dL
Carbon dioxide (CO_2): 21.4 mEq/L
Chloride (Cl-): 105 mEq/L
Calcium (Ca++): 9.4 mg/dL
Uric acid: 1.32 mg/dL
Cholesterol: 158 mg/dL
Red blood cells (RBCs): 2.4 million/uL (mm3)
Hemoglobin (Hbg): 7.8 g/dL
Hematocrit (Hct): 22.3 %

Urine-   Specific gravity: 1.026

3. Nursing History for Elimination Pattern
Bowel

"I had a stool specimen taken a few weeks ago. The doctor said there was no blood in it. I had blood in my stool several years ago. I move my bowels every morning after breakfast and I never take laxatives.

<u>Physical Examination:</u>   Abdomen soft, nontender, nondistended, positive bowel sounds all 4 quadrants. Ability to control anal spincter. No rectal lesions.

<u>Laboratory Findings:</u>   9/3/91

Blood   Stool positive for occult blood
Blood urea nitrogen (BUN): 44 mg/dL

Urine

"I pass my water 8-10 times during the day. I have to go to the bathroom 2 to 3 times during the night. My stream of urine is slower."

The internist observed the stream and noted on the health record a decrease in the force of the urine stream. Client urinated twice during the 20 minute admission assessment.

<u>Physical Examination:</u>	No CVA tenderness. Kidney and bladder examination nonpalpable. No palpable masses.
<u>Laboratory Findings:</u>	9/3/91
Blood-	Creatinine: 1.1 mg/dL
Urine-	Pale yellow, clear. Specific gravity: 1.026. Negative for leukocytes, nitrates, protein, glucose, ketones. Negative white blood cells (WBCs), red blood cells (RBCs), and casts.

4. Nursing History for Activity-Exercise Pattern

"My arthritis is out of control. I am unable to do anything for myself. Please untie my shoes. My hands are swollen and it is hard to move my fingers. I hold onto a chair when I walk around the house. The joints in my legs hurt when I stand or walk. I get tired when I make my breakfast and lunch. My wife opens all the food containers for me before she leaves for work. My feet have been puffy. My blood pressure runs high."

<u>Physical Examination:</u>	Blood pressure (BP): 150/90, pulse (P): 80 regular rhythm, respirations (R) : 20 regular rate. Extremities positive for subcutaneous nodules. Decreased ROM all joints. Abducts 15 degrees both shoulders. Elbow flexion 70 degrees. Right wrist flexion 60 degrees. First and second metacarpophalangeal joints edematous, erythematous, tender and warm to touch. Unable to grasp hand firmly. Left hand in splint. Unable to dress self. Demonstrated unsteady balance and gait when walking. Walked 10 feet to bathroom and sat down twice enroute. Both ankles 2+ edema and erythematous. Positive bunion left foot. No heart palpitations. Lungs clear to auscultation.

Functional Levels

Feeding: 2	Toileting: 2	General mobility: 3
Dressing: 2	Bed mobility: 2	Cooking: 3
Bathing: 2	Home maintenance: 3	Shopping: 3
Grooming: 1		

Functional Level Codes

Level 0: Full self-care
Level 1: Requires use of equipment or device
Level 2: Requires assistance or supervision from another person.
Level 3: Requires assistance or supervision from another person and equipment or device
Level 4: Is dependent and does not participate

Scale for Describing Edema

1 +: Barely detectable	3 +: Indentation of 5 to 10 mm
2 +: Indentation of less than 5 mm	4 +: Indentation of more than 10 mm

Laboratory Findings:	9/3/91
Blood-	Erythrocyte sedimentation rate (ESR) 59 mm/h
	Rheumatoid arthritis factor 1:250 (latex fixation)
X-ray Findings:	Narrowing of joint space and bony erosions visualized.

5. Nursing History for Sleep-Rest Pattern

"At home, I cannot sleep. I hurt all over. I get up in the morning and have difficulty moving. My wife helps me to a standing position. I have no energy. I do not believe in sleeping pills. I take two ecotrin pills before I go to bed. I take an hour nap about 5pm each day after all my business calls have stopped. My eyes feel tired. I am just too tired to talk."

Physical Examination: Stooped posture. Ptosis of eyelids. Dark circles under eyes. Yawning throughout interview. Mispronounces words.

6. Nursing History for Cognitive-Perceptual Pattern

"I am unable to taste or smell anything because of a reaction to my medication, methotrexate. I stopped taking methotrexate two weeks ago. I still cannot taste or smell, and the sores in my mouth hurt."

"My arthritis flares up several times a year and is usually relieved with ecotrin. This time, the pain was not relieved with ecotrin. During the past two weeks the pain has been worse than in the past 30 years. I usually have a dull constant ache in all my joints. It feels like a knife is stabbing each joint. It hurts when you move my joints." Client taught to rate pain on a scale of 0 - 10. "I rate my pain an 8." Facial grimacing and moaning when each joint tested for ROM. I take ecotrin 325 mg, 2 tablets four times a day to relieve my pain, and Tylenol #3 if I still hurt. I took Tylenol #3, 2 tablets at 11 pm last night. Sometimes I get heartburn from taking too much ecotrin." Oriented to time, place and person (oriented x3).

Physical Examination: Hearing: WNL. No ringing in the ears. Wears reading glasses. Conjunctiva pink, moist. Cornea negative scleral icterus. Pupils equal, round, react to light and accommodation (PERRLA.) Nasal mucosa moist. Unable to identify smell on alcohol sponge when eyes closed. Unable to identify the taste of coffee. Lesions present oral cavity.

Laboratory Findings:	9/3/91
Blood·	Salicylate level: 23 mg/dL

Pain rating Intensity scale

0 = no pain	4 = mild pain	8 = disabling pain
1 = slight pain	5 = moderate pain	9 = disabling pain
2 = slight pain	6 = moderate pain	10= Unbearable pain
3 = mild pain	7 = disabling pain	

7. Nursing History for Self-Perception/Self-Concept Pattern

"I am unable to run my photography business. Today, I worked four hours answering the telephone. I was a track star in college and prided myself on my physical fitness. Now look at me. My body is bent over and my joints are large. I am not the man I use to be. I cannot concentrate today." Spoke in halting low voice. Nurse repeated interview questions as client easily distracted. Looked at floor or wall during the interview. Stooped posture with little movement of body. Behavior rated a 2 on a scale of (1) passive to (5) assertive.

8.   Nursing History for Role-Relationship Pattern

"My wife earns the money now and pays all our bills. She works full-time as a secretary. I use to earn all the money. I feel badly about my wife working because she is getting old. She also cares for me. Our children call and visit at least every week. I have 3 sons and 2 daughters. They all help with my photography business and with the maintenance of the house. They have their own homes and families. I do not know how much longer they can help me."

Wife stated "I love to work. I was home caring for our children for 20 years. My husband needs to accept the fact that he cannot work anymore."

Wife accompanied client on admission. Wife holding client's hand during interview. Social worker's note on chart stated, "Observed husband and wife in problem solving situation at home. Wife alert to the needs of husband. Children willingly assist with the business and chores."

9. Nursing History for Sexuality-Reproductive Pattern

"We have 5 children, and had no problems with our sex life when we were young. I lost my interest in sexual relations about five years ago. I am too tired and my joints hurt. I never asked my wife if this bothered her." Staring at floor. No eye contact with interviewer. Mumbling responses.

Physical Examination: Penis, urethra, scrotum, testes, epididymis, inguinal canal within normal limits (WNL). No masses. Prostrate not enlarged. No penile drainage.

10. Nursing History for Coping-Stress Tolerance Pattern

"It took me 10 years before I accepted the fact that I had rheumatoid arthritis. I pace myself during the day. I answer the phone and book appointments for portraits and weddings. I realized a few years ago that I could no longer take wedding pictures so my oldest son does the weddings on the weekends. My children help out with the business. My oldest son is considering giving up his job at an automobile company and taking over the business for me. I can always act as a consultant. I do not smoke or drink anymore. I perform isometric exercises if I feel tense. Right now, I am worried about this infection and my joint pain. I rate my anxiety level a 2 on a scale of 0-5." No wringing hands or diaphoresis. Sitting quietly on bed. Facial muscles taut. Demonstrated isometric exercises. Social worker's note from home visit stated, "Children visit daily. Supportive family structure."

Anxiety Rating Scale		
0 = No anxiety	2 = Increased level of concern	4 = Sympatho-adrenal response
1 = Verbalizes apprehension	3 = Unfocused apprehension	5 = Panic

11.   Nursing History for Value Belief Pattern

"My wife and I have belonged to the same Baptist church for our entire marriage. We go to church each Sunday, no matter how much my joints may be hurting. My faith in God has helped me through some painful days. We attend the potluck dinners on Friday nights and enjoy the fellowship. Our children and their families attend the church. It is wonderful seeing our 10 grandchildren. I assist with the food pantry on Saturdays and give food to folks in need. I enjoy helping other people." Bible on bedside stand. Get-well cards taped to wall. Chaplain's pamphlet lying on bed. Smiled when talking about helping others.

Case Study #2: Human Response to a Surgical Problem: (Carcinoma left breast, Stage I)

DEMOGRAPHIC DATA

Date of Interview: 9/3/91, 11am
Client: Mrs. Judy Smith
Address: 1621 Hampton, Seminole, Florida 34642
Telephone: 339-6341
Contact: Husband
Address of contact: Same as client
Age: 49   Sex: Female   Race: White
Educational background: Associate degree in medical records
Religion: Catholic   Marital status: Married
Usual occupation: Medical record technician for a hospital.
Source of income: Salary from employment. Husband is an accountant.
Insurance: Health Alliance Plan (HAP)
Source of information: Client
Reliability of historian (1-4): 4

ASSESSMENT OF DOENGES AND MOORHOUSE'S DIAGNOSTIC DIVISIONS

1. Nursing History for Activity-Rest Division

"I work full-time as a medical records technician at a hospital. I play tennis once a week. I walk about 2 miles each evening. I usually sleep 8 hours each night. Sometimes I take a 15 minute rest when I arrive home from work. Since I received the biopsy results 2 months ago, I only sleep 2-3 hours. I usually get up and read the newspaper. The doctor ordered sleeping medication for me. I am tired at work lately. My eyelids feel heavy."

Physical Examination:	Slight hand tremor. Firm muscle tone. Lethargic. Oriented to time, place and person. Dark circles under eyes. Rubbing eyes during interview. Ptosis eyelids. Decreased attention span. Gait steady. Yawning throughout interview. Posture well balanced. Full range of motion (ROM). No dyspnea upon exertion. Changed position from bed to chair 5 times during interview.
Medication	Temazepam 30 mg Tab 1 (o) qhs prn

2. Nursing History for Circulation Division

"My usual blood pressure is 120/80. My head has been pounding the past 2 weeks. My heart feels like it is racing. This is a new feeling as I have had no cardiac problems, no chest pain, no heart flutters or racing of my heart in the past. My father has coronary artery disease. I never had rheumatic fever, phlebitis, numbness, tingling or pain in my legs. No, I have had no spitting up of blood, and there has been no change in frequency or amount of urine." Denies chest pain, palpitations or tachycardia.

Medical record reveals previous yearly physical examinations from 1986-1991; blood pressure readings of 120/80, pulse 78, respirations 16.

<u>Physical Examination</u>:   Blood pressure (BP) 150/80 sitting; 146/80 lying. Apical rate 90 regular rhythm at rest. Respirations 24 regular rate. No pedal edema. No shortness of breath (SOB), dyspnea. Wheezing upon expiration. No jugular vein distention. Blanching sign: immediate capillary refill nail beds. Conjunctiva transparent. Sclera white. Extremities warm to the touch.

<u>Peripheral Pulses</u>:
Temporal-4 bilateral
Carotid-4 bilateral
Brachial-4 bilateral
Radial-4 bilateral
Femoral-4 bilateral
Popliteal-4 bilateral
Posterior tibial-4 bilateral
Dorsalis pedis-4 bilateral

Peripheral Pulse Scale

0-Absent	3-Slightly diminished
1-Markedly diminished	4-Normal
2-Moderately diminished	

<u>Diagnostic Studies</u>:

Electrocardiogram- (ECG)   Normal sinus rhythm

Chest x-ray-   Clear lung fields

<u>Laboratory Findings</u>:   9/3/91

Blood-   SGOT: 20 U/L

3. Nursing History for Elimination Division

"I have a bowel movement after dinner each day. I have a problem with constipation for the past 2 months. I decided to take metamucil every night. The doctor prescribed colace once a day. My last bowel movement was last night and the stool was hard. I have stopped eating salads at lunch and dinner. I am too nauseated. My internist does a rectal exam at my annual physical. "I usually urinate 6 times a day. I have no problem with bladder infections. No, I do not have pain or discomfort when I urinate. I never get up at night to urinate."

Medical record reveals no previous problem with constipation as noted on the client's history and physical examinations, 1986-1990.

<u>Physical Examination</u>:   Abdomen nontender, moderately distended, positive bowel sounds all quadrants. Rectal deferred. No CVA tenderness. No palpable masses. Kidney and bladder nonpalpable. Genitalia examination deferred.

Laboratory Findings:	9/3/91
Blood-	Blood urea nitrogen (BUN): 15 mg/dL
Urine-	Amber colored, clear. Specific gravity: 1.025. Negative leucocytes, nitrates, protein, glucose, ketones. Negative for WBCs, RBCs and casts.
Bowel-	Stool specimen negative occult blood. Hard, formed, brown colored stool.
Medications:	Colace: 100 mg (o) qd prn

4. Nursing History for Emotional Reactions Division

"I am not concerned about money but I am concerned about my radical mastectomy scheduled for tomorrow. I hope I can wear a bikini after this surgery. My husband thinks I have a great figure. I told my husband about my surgery but he will not talk about it. We travel a lot and I think he is afraid our trips will be cancelled by my surgery. He will be here shortly. I am a Catholic and have gone to church every Sunday for years. I asked my priest why did I have to get cancer? He did not respond. I believe that God is punishing me for something. This is not fair. I have lived a good life. I told my husband that I would not go to church anymore. I rate my anxiety level a 2 on scale 0-5."

Physical Examination:	Speaking in a loud abrupt voice. Constantly talking. Eyes darting around the room. Facial muscles taut. Face flushed. BP 150/80. P 90. R 24.

Anxiety Rating Scale

0 = No anxiety	2 = Increased level of concern	4 = Sympatho-adrenal response
1 = Verbalizes apprehension	3 = Unfocused apprehension	5 = Panic

5. Nursing History for Food-Fluid Division

"I eat 3 balanced meals a day. I drink 2 juice glasses of water a day. I pack a lunch for work. I buy all the groceries and cook all the meals. My husband does not help. I feel nauseated and too upset to eat today. I have lost 10 pounds in the past 3 weeks. I ate a bowl of soup for dinner at 6pm last night. In the past month, I have had heartburn at least once a day. I do not have food allergies. I do no use diuretics. I feel chilly."

Ate 25% of food on lunch tray. Full pitcher of water on bedside stand.

Typical Daily Intake:

Breakfast-	1 glass orange juice, 1 cup coffee and 1 wheat toast with jam.
Lunch-	Ham on white bread, cookies and 2 cups of coffee.
Dinner-	Steak, baked potato, rolls, butter, chocolate cake and 2 cups coffee.
Evening snack-	Candy

Physical Examination:	Actual height 5'6". Actual weight 110 lbs. Small frame. Temperature 99.2F. Pulse 90. Skin warm to the touch. Skin turgor: shape returned in 10 seconds. No breaks in skin. Hair evenly distributed. Scalp hair texture. Nail beds pink. Positive blanching sign. Teeth: No dentures or partial plates. Oral cavity: lips, breath, tongue, tonsils, pharynx, speech and salivary gland within normal limits (WNL). No difficulty swallowing.

Laboratory Findings:	9/3/91
Blood-	Serum albumin: 5.2 g/dL
	Serum glucose: 105 mg/dL
	Blood urea nitrogen (BUN): 8 mg/dL
	Sodium (Na+): 150 mEq/L
	Chloride (Cl-): 90 mEq/L
	Potassium: 3.0 mEq/L
	Calcium (Ca++): 8.5 mg/dL
	Hemoglobin (Hbg): 11 g/dL
	Hematocrit: 50%
	White blood cells (WBC): 9,000 uL (mm3)
	Red blood cells (RBCs): 4.1 million uL (mm3)
	Prothrombin 13 seconds

6. Nursing History for Hygiene

"I shower and wash my hair every day. I scrub my teeth after every meal."

Physical Examination:	No body odor. Skin clean, hair and nails clean. Skin pale, moist. Hair combed neatly. Nails manicured.

Functional Levels

Feeding: 0	Toileting: 0	General mobility: 0
Dressing: 0	Bed mobility: 0	Cooking: 0
Bathing: 0	Home maintenance: 0	Shopping: 0
Grooming: 0		

Functional Level Codes

Level 0: Full self-care
Level 1: Requires use of equipment or device
Level 2: Requires assistance or supervision from another person.
Level 3: Requires assistance or supervision from another person and
equipment or device
Level 4: Is dependent and does not participate

7. Nursing History for Neurologic Division

"I have had migraine headaches for the past 20 years. I get a migraine once a month. My name is Judy Smith. It is Monday, September 3, 1991. I am at the Urban Hospital. I wear glasses at work to read fine print." Physicians' note stated client has been treated for migraine headaches on outpatient basis at Urban Hospital for past 10 years

Physical Examination: Alert. Pupils equal round react to light and accommodation (PERRLA).
                            No facial drooping. Handgrasps equal. Speech clear. Learns quickly.
                            Ability to read newsprint with glasses. Hears whispered, spoken words.
                            Oriented to time, place and person (oriented x3). Ability to verbalize
                            recent and past events. Denies problems with swallowing.

8. Nursing History for Pain Division

"I have no pain or tenderness in my left breast. I am having a migraine headache right now. It is a steady throbbing pain around my left eye. I rate the intensity a 7 on scale of 0 to 10. I take ergotamine 1 tablet when my headache begins and it usually works. I forgot to bring my ergotamine with me and I need some medication. I get a migraine when I have been under a lot of stress. I get nauseated with the headaches and feel nauseated right now."

Client turned lights off in room. Shades on window pulled. Lying quietly in bed when interviewer arrived in room with eyes closed. Rubbing forehead over left eye. Radio and television off.

Physical Examination: Facial grimacing. Skin pale, moist. Palpable neck and shoulder
                            muscles. Hard irregular, poorly delineated, nonmobile lump felt left
                            upper outer sector breast.

Medications: Ergotamine 2mg (o) onset migraine

Pain rating intensity scale		
0 = no pain	4 = mild pain	8 = disabling pain
1 = slight pain	5 = moderate pain	9 = disabling pain
2 = slight pain	6 = moderate pain	10= Unbearable pain
3 = mild pain	7 = disabling pain	

9. Nursing History for Relationship Alterations Division

"I have been married 27 years. My husband is 52 years old. He works full-time as an accountant. I have worked full-time for 10 years. We have two children ages 21 and 23. Our children are both in college and visit on holidays. We talk with them each weekend on the telephone. I love my husband and children. My husband and I live in a ranch home in a small town. Our social life consists of attending office parties at our places of employment and church functions. My father lives 25 miles from my house and joins us for Sunday dinners. I hope this surgery will not change my relationship with my husband. I am so nervous. I wish my husband would hurry up and get here. At home, I go for walks just to get rid of all my anger."

Husband not present. Smiled when talking about husband and children. Began crying during interview. Wringing hands. Began pacing floor.

10. Nursing History for Safety Division

"I fell on the tennis court in 1985 and broke my left wrist and arm. I have no problems with hearing."

Physical Examination: Temperature 99.2 F (o). Intact skin integrity. One inch scar on left
                            breast. Strength equal all extremities. Muscle tone firm. ROM wrist
                            within normal limits.

11. Nursing History for Sexuality - Female Division

"I started menstruating at 13 years and my periods last 3 days. My last period was August 25, 1991. I do not have any vaginal discharge. I had 2 pregnancies and 2 children. I use oral contraceptives. I noticed the lump in my left breast during my monthly self-breast examination six months ago. I kept putting off going to the doctor. Finally, I went to the doctor 2 months ago. A biopsy was performed at that time. The doctor told me the tumor was malignant. I go to surgery tomorrow to have my left breast removed. The doctor said he might take some nodes out. I had been very healthy until this happened to me. I had a mammogram and a pap smear every year for the past 5 years. I am concerned my husband will find me unattractive after this mastectomy. We use to have sex at least once a week. Now, we rarely have sex. My husband says he is too tired and does not want to talk about sex. Sex is not the most important thing. I know he loves me as he is thoughtful."

Frown on face when discussing sexual relations.

Physical Examination: Left breast lump palpable, nontender, dimpling of skin over upper outer sector. Hard, irregular, poorly delineated, non mobile lump. No nipple discharge. No palpable lumps in right breast. No vaginal drainage or lesions.

Biopsy: 7/3/91. Left breast biopsy positive for primary tumor stage T1.

Mammogram: 7/3/91. Tumor 2 cm with no fixation to under lying pectoral fascia and/or muscle.

TNM Clinical Staging of Breast Carcinoma

Stage 1: Tumor-less than 2 cm in diameter
Nodes-negative
Metastases-no distant metastases

Stage 2: Tumor-greater than 2 cm and less than 5 cm in diameter
Nodes-negative if no nodes present; positive if nodes present and are fixed to one another or to to other structures
Metastases-no distant metastases

Stage 3: Tumor-greater than 5 cm or tumor of any size with direct extension to the chest wall
Nodes-supraclavicular or infraclavicular involvement
Metastases- no distant metastases

Stage 4: Tumor-tumor of any size
Nodes-positive or negative
Metastases-distant metastases present

---

12. Nursing History for Teaching-Learning Division

"I have an associate degree in medical records. Learning new things has been easy for me. My father is alive, 75 years old, and has coronary artery disease. My last physical examination was 2 months ago. I have a dental examination every 6 months. I drink 5 cups of coffee per day and more when I get nervous. I do not drink alcohol or use recreational drugs."

"I expect to be cured of cancer after this surgery. I am not worried even though my maternal grandmother died of breast cancer at age 49 and my mother died of breast cancer at age 53. I anticipate no problems. This will be a quick surgery and recovery period. I plan to be home 2 days after my mastectomy and return to work 2 weeks from the day of surgery. My church group said they would bring dinners over for the first week after discharge."

Dominant language English. Not observed drinking coffee. Wringing hands.

<u>Admitting diagnosis:</u>   Carcinoma left breast, Stage I.

<u>Current medications:</u>

   Prescription-   Colace 100 mg (o) bid

   Nonprescription-   Metamucil 1 Tbsp. prn

13. Nursing History for Ventilation Division

"I have hay fever and if it gets bad, I develop asthma. I wheeze when I have an asthma attack and get short of breath. My mother and maternal grandmother had asthma. My eyes and nose have been itching and watering this week. I take benadryl for my hay fever and took benadryl 25 mg before I came to the hospital today. I also took 2 whiffs of alupent in my nebulizer this morning because I started to sound wheezy The alupent stopped the wheezing sounds for a few hours. I do not want my asthma to begin especially since I will be going to surgery. I have never smoked."

<u>Physical Examination:</u>   Respirations 24, regular rate, rhythm. No nasal flaring or use of accessory muscles. Redness and lacrimation (tearing) eyes. Nasal turbinates pale, edematous, and watery nasal drainage. Auscultation chest revealed minimal wheezing on expiration both lungs. Temperature 99.2F. (o). No smoking observed.

<u>Chest x-ray:</u>   Negative

<u>Skin test:</u>   Positive allergens for grass

<u>Current Medications:</u>
   Prescription-   Benadryl 25 mg (o) q6h prn
                             Alupent 0.65mg 2 inhalations q4h prn

PART II: DEFINING THE STEPS IN THE NURSING PROCESS

DEFINITION

The nursing process is a systematic method of assessing human responses to health problems and developing written nursing care plans aimed at resolving the problems. The health problems may be related to the client, family, significant other or the community. The nursing process documents the nurse's contribution to the reduction or resolution of the client's problems.

The nurse strives to resolve health problems through the application of the five step nursing process:

STEP 1: ASSESSMENT
STEP 2: NURSING DIAGNOSIS
STEP 3: PLANNING
STEP 4: IMPLEMENTATION
STEP 5: EVALUATION

The five steps are graphically depicted in the nursing process cycle (Figure 2-1). The nursing process cycle begins when the client enters the healthcare delivery system. The nurse initiates the first step of the cycle, assessment, by gathering data from the client. A nursing diagnosis related to the client's problem is identified in the second step. Within the third step, the nurse and client work together to formulate a plan of action aimed at resolution of the client's problem. The plan includes establishment of outcome criteria and nursing orders (interventions). During the fourth step, the plan is implemented by the nurse and the client. In the fifth step, the client and the nurse evaluate whether the outcome criteria have been achieved, and the problem resolved. The client exits the cycle if the outcome criteria are achieved. The client reenters the cycle if the outcome criteria have not been achieved. The nurse reassesses the client and plan to determine the factors affecting outcome criteria achievement.

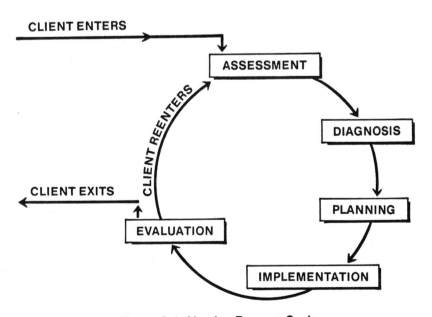

Figure 2-1: Nursing Process Cycle

Step 1: Assessment

PURPOSE

The purpose of the assessment step is to gather information and establish a data base for the client. The client is assessed upon entry into a healthcare delivery system.

COMPONENTS OF THE ASSESSMENT STEP

1. Data Collection
2. Data Validation
3. Pattern or Division Identification

1. Data Collection: *What information does the nurse need to know?*

Data collection is the systematic gathering of information about the client including client strengths and weaknesses. Data is collected from the client, family, significant other, community, charts and records. The client is the primary source of information, the original provider of data. Secondary sources of information consist of data that already exist or from individuals other than the client. Secondary sources include the client's health record, reports of laboratory and diagnostic tests, family, significant other, community and health team members.

Major methods of collecting data are observation, interview, consultation and examination.

Data Collection Methods

Observation: A data collection method in which data are collected through visual observations.

Interview: A method of data collection in which the interviewer, the nurse, obtains responses from a client. obtains responses from a client in a face-to-face encounter.

Consultation: A specialist is sought to identify ways to treat and manage client problems.

Examination: The process of inspection of the body and its systems to determine the presence or absence of disease based on the following findings.
Physical: Four procedures utilized are inspection, palpation, percussion and auscultation.
Laboratory: Urinalysis, blood tests and cultures.
X-rays: Visualization of body spaces, and their function.

Human beings respond differently to problems. For example, the cultural values, beliefs and religious practices of clients may differ. It is essential for the nurse to assess the client's individual response to a problem and avoid generalizations.

The data collected forms the client's data baseline. The baseline data will be used for future comparison of the client's values and standards to ascertain the effectiveness of treatment, nursing care and the achievement of outcome criteria. During data collection, the clinical data are categorized as subjective or objective.

Subjective Data

Subjective data refers to the client's perceptions and sensations about a health problem. The client expresses subjective perceptions and feelings such as self-worth or pain. Subjective data is information the client tells the nurse during the nursing assessment interview, that is, the comments the nurse hears. Subjective data can be called symptoms. Subjective data or symptoms are phenomena experienced by a client and may be a departure from client's normal sensations.

Examples of Subjective Data

"I have a headache."	"I hurt all over."	"I feel sad."
"I feel short of breath."	"My legs feel weak."	"I feel hot."
"My stomach is burning."	"I feel hot."	"I feel tired."

The above examples illustrate the subjective data that a client may express to the nurse. Headache, nausea, burning, fatigue, stiffness, shortness of breath, warmth, dizziness and sadness are sensations the client feels. These feelings are not necessarily visible to the nurse. Clients verbalize their feelings to the nurse.

Exercise A: Identification of Subjective Data

The purpose of Exercise A is to aid in identifying the subjective data presented by the client. Fill in the blanks with subjective data noted in case study #1, p. 7-12. Examples of subjective data have been cited from case study #1 for each functional health pattern.

•Pattern #1: Health Perception-Health Management p. 7

1. "My knuckles are swollen." _____

2. _____
   _____

3. _____
   _____

4. _____
   _____

5. _____
   _____

6. _____
   _____

7. _____
   _____

8. _____
   _____

•Pattern #2: Nutritional-Metabolic p. 8

1. "I sweat a lot." _____

2. _____
   _____

3. _____
   _____

4. _____
   _____

5. _____
   _____

6. _____
   _____

•Pattern #3: Elimination p. 9

1. "I had blood in my stool several years ago." _____

2. _____

   _____

3. _____

   _____

•Pattern #4: Activity-Exercise p. 10

1. "I cannot do anything for myself." _____

2. _____

   _____

3. _____

   _____

4. _____

   _____

5. _____

   _____

6. _____

   _____

7. _____

   _____

•Pattern #5: Sleep-Rest p. 11

1. "My eyes feel tired." _____

2 _____

   _____

3. _____

   _____

4. _____

   _____

•Pattern #6: Cognitive-Perceptual p. 11

1. "I hurt in all my joints." _____

2. _____
   _____

3. _____
   _____

4. _____
   _____

5. _____
   _____

•Pattern #7: Self-Perception/Self-Concept p. 11

1. "I am not the man I used to be." _____

2. _____
   _____

3. _____
   _____

4. _____
   _____

5. _____
   _____

•Pattern #8: Role-Relationship p. 12

1. "My wife earns the money now...she cares for me." _____

2. _____
   _____

3. _____
   _____

•Pattern #9: Sexuality-Reproductive p. 12

1. "I lost my interest in sex five years ago." _____

2. _____
   _____

•Pattern #10: Coping-Stress Tolerance p. 12

1. "I pace myself during the day." _____

2. _____

   _____

3. _____

   _____

4. _____

   _____

•Pattern #11: Value-Belief p. 12

1. "My faith in God has helped me." _____

2. _____

   _____

3. _____

   _____

4. _____

   _____

Exercise B: Identification of Subjective Data

The purpose of Exercise B is to aid in identifying the subjective data presented by the client. Fill in the blanks with subjective data noted in case study #2, p. 13-19. Examples of subjective data from case study #2 have been cited for each diagnostic division.

•Diagnostic Division #1: Activity-Rest p. 13

1. "I am tired at work lately." _____

2. _____

3. _____

4. _____

5. _____

6. _____

7. _____

•Diagnostic Division #2: Circulation p. 13

1. "My blood pressure runs 120/80." _____

2. _____

3. _____

•Diagnostic Division #3: Elimination p. 14

1. "I have a problem with constipation." _____

2. _____

3. _____

•Diagnostic Division #4: Emotional Reactions p. 15

1. "I am concerned about my mastectomy tomorrow." _____

2. _____

_____

3. _____

_____

4. _____

_____

5. _____

_____

6. _____

_____

•Diagnostic Division #5: Food-Fluid p. 15

1. "I feel chilly." _____

2. _____

_____

3. _____

_____

4. _____

_____

5. _____

_____

•Diagnostic Division #6: Hygiene p. 16

1. "I shower each day." _____

2. _____

_____

3. _____

_____

•Diagnostic Division #7: Neurologic p. 16

1. "I wear glasses to read the newspaper." _____

2. _____
   _____

3. _____
   _____

•Diagnostic Division #8: Pain p. 17

1. "I am having a migraine headache right now." _____

2. _____
   _____

3. _____
   _____

4. _____
   _____

5. _____
   _____

•Diagnostic Division #9: Relationship Alterations p. 17

1. "I wish my husband would hurry up and get here." _____

2. _____
   _____

3. _____
   _____

4. _____
   _____

5. _____
   _____

•Diagnostic Division #10: Safety p. 17

1. "In 1985, I fell and broke my left wrist and arm." _____

•Diagnostic Division #11: Sexuality-Female p. 18

1. "The doctor told me the tumor was malignant." _____

2. _____

   _____

3. _____

   _____

4. _____

   _____

•Diagnostic Division #12: Teaching-Learning p. 18

1. "I drink 5 cups of coffee every day." _____

2. _____

   _____

3. _____

   _____

4. _____

   _____

•Diagnostic Division #13: Ventilation p. 19

1. "I have hay fever." _____

2. _____

   _____

3. _____

   _____

Objective Data

Objective data is based on observable phenomena and presented factually. The observed phenomena is gathered by someone other than the client. The objective data may be observed or measured. Objective data is information collected through the nurse's senses. Objective data is information that the nurse can: (a) see (observation) (inspection), (b) feel (palpation), (c) hear (auscultation) (percussion) or (d) smell. Objective data can be called signs.

Definitions:

Observation:	Looking at the client and reporting what the nurse saw.
Inspection:	The visual examination of the external surface of the body, movements and posture.
Palpation:	The process of examining by application of the hands or fingers to the external surface of the body to detect evidence of abnormalities in the various organs.
Auscultation:	The process of listening for sounds within the body, usually to sounds of thoracic or abdominal viscera to detect abnormalities. A stethoscope is used.
Percussion:	Use of the fingers to tap the body lightly and sharply to determine position, size and consistency of an underlying structure and the presence of fluid or pus in a cavity.

Examples of Objective Data

Observation:	Nasal flaring. Facial grimacing. Respirations 30, shallow. Hemoglobin (Hbg) 7.8 g/dL Serum potassium (K+) 2.5 mEq/L
Palpation:	Bladder palpable. Tenderness right lower quadrant (RLQ) abdomen.
Auscultation:	Crackling sounds right lower lobe (RLL) lung. Borborygmi all quadrants abdomen.
Percussion:	Dullness right lower lobe (RLL) of the lung. Dullness right lower quadrant (RLQ) abdomen.

The above examples illustrate the objective data a client may display to the nurse. Nasal flaring can be seen, organs palpated, breath sounds heard and the resonance and pitch of sound projected from percussion can be heard.

Exercise C: Identification of Objective Data

The purpose of Exercise C is to assist in identifying objective data demonstrated by the client. Fill in the blanks with objective data from case study #1, p. 7-12. Examples of objective data from case study #1 have been cited for each functional health pattern.

● **Pattern #1: Health Perception-Health Management p. 7**

1. Edema right first and second metacarpal phalanges

2. _____

3. _____

4. _____

5. _____

6. _____

7. _____

8. _____

● **Pattern #2: Nutritional-Metabolic p. 8**

1. Skin turgor: shape returned in 15 seconds

2. _____

3. _____

4. _____

5. _____

6. _____

•Pattern #3: Elimination   p. 9

1. 9/3/91 No melena in stool specimen

2. _____

_____

3. _____

_____

•Pattern #4:   Activity-Exercise   p. 10

1. 70 degree elbow flexion

2. _____

_____

3. _____

_____

4. _____

_____

5. _____

_____

6. _____

_____

7. _____

_____

•Pattern #5: Sleep-Rest   p. 11

1. Ptosis of eyelids

2. _____

_____

3. _____

_____

4. _____

_____

•Pattern #6: Cognitive-Perceptual   p.11

1. Facial grimacing. _____

2. _____

_____

3. _____

_____

4. _____

_____

5. _____

_____

•Pattern #7: Self-Perception/Self-Concept p. 11

1. Spoke in halting low voice. _____

2. _____

_____

3. _____

_____

4. _____

_____

5. _____

_____

•Pattern #8: Role-Relationship   p. 12

1. Wife holding client's hand during interview. _____

2. _____

_____

3. _____

_____

•Pattern #9: Sexuality-Reproductive p. 12

1. Mumbling responses to questions _____

2. _____

_____

•Pattern #10: Coping-Stress Tolerance p. 12

1. Paces energy level. _____

2. _____
   _____

3. _____
   _____

4. _____
   _____

•Pattern #11: Value-Belief p. 12

1. Bible on bedside stand. _____

2. _____
   _____

3. _____
   _____

4. _____
   _____

Exercise D: Identification of Objective Data

The purpose of Exercise D is to assist in identifying objective data demonstrated by the client. Fill in the blanks with objective data from case study #2, p. 13-19. Examples of objective data from case study #2 have been cited for each diagnostic division.

•Division #1: Activity-Rest p. 13

1. Slight hand tremor. _____

2. _____
   _____

3. _____
   _____

4. _____
   _____

5. _____
   _____

6. _____
   _____

•Division #2: Circulation p. 13

1. Actual blood pressure 150/90 mm Hg _____

2. _____
   _____

3. _____
   _____

•Division #3: Elimination p. 14

1. Hard, formed, brown colored stool. _____

2. _____
   _____

3. _____
   _____

•Division #4: Emotional Reactions p. 15

1. Facial muscles taut. _____

2. _____
   _____

3. _____
   _____

4. _____
   _____

5. _____
   _____

6. _____
   _____

• Division #5: Food-Fluid p. 15

1. Skin warm to touch. _____

2. _____
   _____

3. _____
   _____

4. _____
   _____

5. _____
   _____

•Division #6: Hygiene p. 16

1. Skin clean. _____

2. _____
   _____

•Division #7: Neurologic p. 16

1. Ability to read newsprint with glasses. _____

2. _____
   _____

3. _____
   _____

•Division #8: Pain p. 17

1. Facial grimacing. _____

2. _____
   _____

3. _____
   _____

4. _____
   _____

5. _____
   _____

•Division #9: Relationship Alterations p. 17

1. Husband not present. _____
   _____

2. _____
   _____

3. _____
   _____

4. _____
   _____

5. _____
   _____

•Division #10: Safety p. 17

1. Wrist 80-90 degree flexion and extension _____

•Division #11: Sexuality-Female p. 18

1. Left breast biopsy positive primary tumor stage T1 _____

2. _____
   _____

3. _____
   _____

4. _____
   _____

•Division #12: Teaching-Learning   p. 18

1. Drank 500-750 mg caffeine in coffee per day. _____

2. _____

   _____

3. _____

   _____

4. _____

   _____

•Division #13: Ventilation   p. 19

1. Minimal wheezing upon expiration. _____

2. _____

   _____

3. _____

   _____

4. _____

   _____

2. Data Validation: *Does the client data reflect normal or abnormal values and standards? Does the objective data confirm and support the subjective data? Is the information collected accurate?*

Data validation is the comparison of data, subjective and objective, gathered from primary (client) and secondary sources (e.g., health record) with accepted normal standards and values. A standard or value is an accepted rule or measure.

The nurse compares the client's comments, subjective data, with the client's objective measurable data. The nurse verifies if the objective data validates the subjective data. The nurse checks if the client's values, subjective and objective, fall within the range of accepted normal standards and values. The nurse compares the client's data to a wide range of objective measurable standards and values, such as normal vital signs, laboratory values, diagnostic tests, basic food groups, normal growth and development.

References document accepted standards and values for laboratory findings, diagnostic tests, physical examinations and behaviors (See Appendices H-L, p. 163-174) for examples of accepted normal standards and values for use in Exercises E and F, p. 45-59).

In the following example, the client values fail to fall within the range of accepted normal values.

Examples of Data Validation

Subjective Data	Objective Data	Normal Values
"My legs feel weak"	Serum K+ 2.5mEq/L	Serum K+ 3.0-5/3 mEq/L
"My blood pressure is usually 110/70."	Blood pressure 170/90 mmHg	Blood pressure 120/80 mmHg
"I feel tired all the time."	Hb 9.0 g/dL	Female Hb: 12.0-16.0 g/dL Male Hb: 3.5-18.0 g/dL

Exercise E: Data Validation

The purpose of Exercise E is to learn to compare gathered data with accepted normal standards and values to determine the client's abnormal values. Listed below are subjective data validated by objective data gathered from case study #1. Compare the client's subjective and objective values to accepted normal standards and values. A list of accepted normal values necessary to complete Exercise E are located in Appendices H-L, p. 163-174. A comparison of the subjective and objective data to accepted normal values has been cited from case study #1.

•Pattern #1: Health Perception/Management SD: p. 25, OD: p. 35

1. Client Value:
SD: "My knuckles are swollen."
OD: Edema right first and second metacarpal phalanges
Normal value: No edema metacarpal joints

2. Client Value:
SD: "...pain...swelling, redness, warmth over knuckles."
OD: Warmth, redness, edema right metacarpal joints
Normal Value:

3. Client Value:
SD: "I had an infected bunion on my left foot."
OD: Ulcer left foot crusty yellowish rim. Temp. 101F(R)
Normal Value:

4. Client Value:
SD: "I could not taste."
OD: Lesions throughout oral cavity.
Normal Value:

5. Client Value:
SD: "I have felt chills."
OD: Temperature 101 F (R). Diaphoretic. Skin warm touch
Normal Value:

6. Client Value:
SD: "...worse attack of arthritis in past 30 years."
OD: No relief symptoms with cortisone injection 8/18/91
Normal Value:

7. Client Value:
SD: "I am allergic to methotrexate."
OD: 8/12/91 Methotrexate 2.5 mg/qd x5days. D/C 8/18/91
Normal Value:

8. **Client Value:**
    SD: "I have felt pain..."
    OD: Facial grimacing; moaning upon joint movement.
    Normal Value:

●Pattern #2: Nutritional-Metabolic SD: p. 25,   OD: p. 35

1. **Client Value**
    SD: "I sweat a lot."
    OD: Skin turgor: Shape returned in 15 seconds
    Normal Value: Prompt return of skin to normal shape

2. **Client Value:**
    SD: "I feel chilly."
    OD: Temp. 101F (R). Skin hot to touch. Diaphoretic.
    Normal Value:

3. **Client Value:**
    SD: "I have lost weight."
    OD: Weight loss 10 lbs. past 6 months.
    Normal Value:

4. **Client Value:**
    SD: "I drink 2 juice glasses of water a day."
    OD: 24 hour oral fluid intake 930cc
    Normal Value:

5. **Client Value:**
    SD: "I have given up using salt."
    OD: Low sodium, 2 g pureed diet ordered by physician
    Normal Value:

6. **Client Value:**
    SD: "My mouth is full of sores."
    OD: Lesions throughout buccal mucosa.
    Normal Value:

●Pattern #3: Elimination SD: p. 26, OD: p. 36

1. **Client Value:**
    SD: "I had blood in my stool several years ago."
    OD: 9/3/91 No melena in stool specimen
    Normal Value: No melena in stool.

2. Client Value:
SD: "I move my bowels every morning."
OD: Abdomen nondistended, nontender
Normal Value: _____

_____

3. Client Value:
SD: "My stream of urine is slower."
OD: Internist noticed decrease in force urine stream
Normal Value: _____

_____

•Pattern #4: Activity-Exercise SD: p. 26, OD: p. 36

1. Client Value:
SD: "I cannot do anything for myself."
OD: 70 degrees elbow flexion
Normal Value: 150 degree elbow flexion

2. Client Value:
SD: "My hands are swollen...hard to move my fingers"
OD: Weak hand grasp. Swelling metacarpal phalange joints
Normal Value: _____

_____

3. Client Value:
SD: "My feet have been puffy."
OD: Both ankles 2+ edema
Normal Value: _____

_____

4. Client Value:
SD: "My blood pressure runs high."
OD: BP 150/90
Normal Value: _____

_____

5. Client Value:
SD: "I get tired when I make my breakfast and lunch."
OD: Walked 10 feet to bathroom and sat down twice enroute.
Normal Value: _____

_____

6. Client Value
SD: "My wife opens all the food containers..."
OD: Unable to grasp hand firmly.
Normal Value: _____

_____

7. **Client value:**
   SD: "I hold onto a chair when I walk around."
   OD: Unsteady gait and balance when walking.
   Normal Value: _____

   _____

●**Pattern #5: Sleep-Rest SD: p. 26, OD: p. 36**

1. **Client Value:**
   SD: "My eyes feel tired."
   OD: Ptosis of eyelids
   Normal Value: No ptosis (drooping) of eyelids.

2. **Client Value:**
   SD: "I cannot sleep."
   OD: Dark circles under eyes. Ptosis eyelids
   Normal Value: _____

   _____

3. **Client Value:**
   SD: "I have no energy."
   OD: Yawning throughout interview.
   Normal Value: _____

   _____

4. **Client Value:**
   SD: "I am just too tired to talk."
   OD: Mispronounces words.
   Normal Value: _____

   _____

●**Pattern #6: Cognitive-Perceptual SD: p. 27, OD: p. 37**

1. **Client Value:**
   SD: "I hurt in all my joints."
   OD: Facial grimacing
   Normal Value: No joint pain. No facial grimacing.

2. **Client Value:**
   SD: "This time, the pain was not relieved with ecotrin."
   OD: Order for Ecotrin 325 mg 2 tablets 4 times/qd
   Normal Value: _____

   _____

3. **Client Value:**
   SD: "I rate my pain an 8."
   OD: Facial grimacing/moaning when joints tested for ROM
   Normal Value: _____

   _____

4. Client Value:

SD: "It feels like a knife stabbing each joint."

OD: Facial grimacing and moaning upon movement joint

Normal Value:

5. Client Value:

SD: "I cannot taste or smell."

OD: Inability to identify the smell of alcohol and the taste of coffee

Normal Value:

•Pattern #7: Self-Perception/Self-Concept SD: p. 27, OD: p. 37

1. Client Value:

SD: "I am not the man I should be."

OD: Spoke in halting, low voice.

Normal Value: Feelings of self-worth.

2. Client Value:

SD: "My body is bent over and my joints are large."

OD: Stooped posture with little body movement.

Normal Value:

3. Client Value:

SD: "I am unable to run my photography business."

OD: Behavior rated 2.

Normal Value:

4. Client Value:

SD: "Please repeat your questions."

OD: Easily distracted. Interview questions repeated.

Normal Value:

5. Client Value:

SD: "I feel badly about my wife working..."

OD: Looked at floor or wall during interview.

Normal Value:

•Pattern #8: Role-Relationship SD: p. 27, OD: p. 37

1. Client Value:

SD: "My wife earns the money now...she cares for me."

OD: Wife holding client's hand

Normal Value: Caring relationship.

2. Client Value:
SD: "(Children) help with my photography business and with the maintenance of the house."
OD: Social workers noted children assist with business
Normal Value: _____

3. Client Value:
SD: "My husband needs to accept the fact...cannot work"
OD: Wife/client observed in problem solving situation
Normal Value: _____

•Pattern #9: Sexuality-Reproductive SD: p. 27, OD: p. 37

1. Client Value:
SD: "I never asked my wife if it bothered her."
OD: Mumbling responses to questions.
Normal Value: Ability to express self to loved ones.

2. Client Value:
SD: "I am too tired and my joints hurt."
OD: No eye contact with interviewer.
Normal Value: _____

•Pattern #10: Coping-Stress Tolerance SD: p. 28, OD: p. 38

1. Client Value:
SD: "I pace myself during the day."
OD: Paces energy level
Normal Value: Time management to conserve energy.

2. Client Value:
SD: "I am worried about this infection and joint pain."
OD: Facial muscles taut.
Normal Value: _____

3. Client Value:
SD: "It took me 10 years accept the fact that I had rheumatoid arthritis."
OD: No wringing hands. Rated anxiety level 2 scale 0-5
Normal Value: _____

4. Client Value:
SD: "I perform isometric exercises if I feel tense."
OD: Demonstrated isometric exercises.
Normal Value: _____

•Pattern #11: Value-Belief SD: p. 28, OD: p. 38

1. **Client Value:**
   SD: "My faith in God has helped me." _____
   OD: Bible on bedside stand. _____

   Normal Value: Belief system provides meaning to life. _____

2. **Client Value:**
   SD: "I enjoy helping other people." _____
   OD: Many get-well cards posted on the wall. _____

   Normal Value: _____

   _____

3. **Client value:**
   SD: "We go to church every Sunday..." _____
   OD: Chaplain's pamphlet lying on bed. _____

   Normal Value: _____

   _____

4. **Client value:**
   SD: "I work in the food pantry and help those in need." _____
   OD: Smiled when talking about helping others. _____

   Normal Value: _____

   _____

Exercise F: Data Validation

The purpose of Exercise F is to learn to compare gathered data with accepted normal standards and values to determine the client's abnormal values. Listed below are subjective data validated by objective data from case study #2. Compare the client's subjective and objective values to accepted normal standards and values. A list of accepted normal values necessary to complete Exercise F are located in Appendices H-L, p. 163-174. A comparison of subjective and objective data to accepted normal values has been cited from case study #2.

•Division #1: Activity-Rest   SD: p. 29,   OD: p. 39

1. **Client Value:**
   SD: "I am tired at work lately." _____
   OD: Slight hand tremor _____

   Normal Value: No hand tremor _____

2. **Client Value:**
   SD: "I only sleep 2-3 hours." _____
   OD: Dark circles under eyes. _____

   Normal Value: _____
   _____

3. **Client Value:**
   SD: "My eyelids feel heavy." _____
   OD: Ptosis eyelids. _____

   Normal Value: _____
   _____

4. **Client Value:**
   SD: "I usually sleep 8 hours." _____
   OD: Decreased attention span _____

   Normal Value: _____
   _____

5. **Client Value:**
   SD: "The doctor ordered sleeping medication for me." _____
   OD: Temazepam 30 mg Tab. 1 (o) qhs prn ordered _____

   Normal Value: _____
   _____

6. **Client Value:**
   SD: "I am tired at work lately." _____
   OD: Yawning during interview. Slouched posture. _____

   Normal Value: _____
   _____

7. **Client Value:**
   SD: "I walk about 2 miles each evening." _____
   OD: Firm muscle tone. No dyspnea upon exertion. _____

   Normal Value: _____
   _____

•**Division #2:   Circulation SD: p. 29, OD: p. 39**

1. **Client Value:**
    SD: "My usual blood pressure is 120/80."
    OD: Actual BP 150/80 mm Hg
    Normal Value: 120/80 mm Hg

2. **Client Value:**
    SD: "My heart feels like it is racing."
    OD: Pulse 90 at rest
    Normal Value:

3. **Client Value:**
    SD: "My head has been pounding for the past 2 weeks."
    OD: Rubbing forehead over left eye. BP 150/80. Pulse 90
    Normal Value:

•**Division #3: Elimination SD: p. 29, OD: p. 39**

1. **Client Value:**
    SD: "I have a problem with constipation."
    OD: Hard stool
    Normal Value: Formed, moist stool

2. **Client Value:**
    SD: "...take metamucil everyday...take colace once day."
    OD: Abdomen moderately distended. Colace 100 mg qd prn
    Normal Value:

3. **Client Value:**
    SD: "I usually urinate 6 times a day."
    OD: Specific gravity 1.025. Straw colored, clear urine.
    Normal Value:

•**Division #4: Emotional Reactions SD: p. 30, OD: p.40**

1. **Client Value:**
    SD: "I am concerned about my mastectomy tomorrow."
    OD: Facial muscles taut
    Normal Value: Toned, not taut facial muscles

2. **Client value:**
    SD: "I hope I can wear a bikini after this surgery."
    OD: Eyes darting around the room.
    Normal value:

3. Client Value:
SD: "This is not fair."
OD: Speaking in loud abrupt voice.
Normal Value:

4. Client value:
SD: "I believe God is punishing me."
OD: Face flushed.
Normal Value:

5. Client Value:
SD: "I told my husband...I would not go church anymore."
OD: Constantly talking.
Normal Value:

6. Client Value:
SD: "I rate my anxiety level a 2."
OD: Rated anxiety level 2 on scale 0-5.
Normal Value:

•Division #5: Food-Fluid SD: p. 30, OD: p. 40

1. Client Value:
SD: "I feel chilly."
OD: Skin warm to touch
Normal Value: Skin warm to touch

2. Client value:
SD: "I feel nauseated and too upset to eat today."
OD: Ate 25% food on lunch tray.
Normal Value:

3. Client Value:
SD: "I have lost 10 pounds in past 3 weeks."
OD: Actual weight 110 lbs. Height 5'6", small frame.
Normal Value:

4. Client Value:
SD: "I eat 3 balanced meals a day."
OD: Typical daily intake not balanced with 4 food groups.
Normal Value:

5. **Client Value:**
   SD: "I drink 2-3 juice glasses of water a day."
   OD: Skin turgor: shape returned in 10 seconds.
   Normal Value: _____

•Division #6: Hygiene SD: p. 30, OD: p. 40

1. **Client Value:**
   SD: "I shower and wash my hair every day."
   OD: Skin clean. No body odor.
   Normal Value: Daily hygiene

2. **Client Value:**
   SD: "I scrub my teeth after every meal."
   OD: 32 permanent teeth. No plaque. No dentures/plate.
   Normal Value: _____

•Division #7: Neurologic SD: p. 31, OD: p. 40

1. **Client Value:**
   SD: "I wear glasses at work to read the fine print."
   OD: Reads newsprint with glasses
   Normal Value: Reads newsprint without glasses

2. **Client Value:**
   SD: "My name is Judy Smith. It is Monday, September 3. I am at the Urban Hospital"
   OD: Oriented to time, place and person.
   Normal Value: _____

3. **Client Value:**
   SD: "I have had migraine headaches for the past 20 years."
   OD: Physician's note...treated migraine in outpatient department for past 10 years.
   Normal Value: _____

•Division #8: Pain SD: p. 31, OD: p. 41

1. **Client Value:**
   SD: "I am having a migraine headache right now."
   OD: Facial grimacing
   Normal Value: No headaches

2. **Client Value:**
   SD: "It is steady throbbing pain around my left eye."
   OD: Rubbing forehead over left eye. Lights off in room.
   Normal Value: _____

3. Client Value:
SD: "I rate the intensity a 7 on scale 0 to 10."
OD: Palpable neck and shoulder muscles

Normal Value: _____

4. Client Value:
SD: "I do not have any pain in my left breast."
OD: Hard, irregular, poorly delineated, nonmobile lump

Normal Value: _____

5. Client Value:
SD: "...I feel nauseated."
OD: Pale skin.

Normal Value: _____

•Division #9: Relationship Alterations SD: p.31, OD: p.41

1. Client Value:
SD: "I wish my husband would hurry up and get here."
OD: Husband not present
Normal Value: Support from significant other

2. Client Value:
SD: "I am so nervous."
OD: Wringing hands.

Normal Value: _____

3. Client Value:
SD: "I hope this surgery will not hurt our relationship."
OD: Began crying.

Normal Value: _____

4. Client Value:
SD: "I love my husband and children."
OD: Smiled when talking about husband and children.

Normal Value: _____

5. Client Value:
SD: At home, I go for walks to get rid of my anger."
OD: Began pacing floor. Wringing hands.

Normal Value: _____

•Division #10: Safety SD: p. 31, OD: p. 41

1. **Client Value:**
    SD: "In 1985, I fell and broke my left wrist."
    OD: Wrist 80-90 degree flexion and extension
    Normal Value: Wrist 80-90 degree flexion and extension

•Division #11: Sexuality-Female SD: p. 32, OD: p. 41

1. **Client Value:**
    SD: "The doctor told me the tumor was malignant."
    OD: Breast biopsy positive for primary tumor stage T1.
    Normal Value: No breast lumps. No malignancies.

2. **Client Value:**
    SD: "I noticed the lump in my left breast..."
    OD: Demonstrated correct self-breast examination.
    Normal Value: _____

3. **Client Value:**
    SD: "I had a mammogram...every year for past 5 years."
    OD: Diagnostic studies reflect yearly mammogram 1986-1991.
    Normal Value: _____

4. **Client Value:**
    SD: "We use to have sex once a week."
    OD: Frown on face when discussing sexual relationship
    Normal Value: _____

•Division #12: Teaching-Learning SD: p. 32, OD: p. 42

1. **Client Value:**
    SD: "I drink 5 cups of coffee every day."
    OD: Drinks 500-750 mg caffeine per day
    Normal Value: 100-150 mg caffeine/qd; 100-150mg c. coffee

2. **Client Value:**
    SD: "I expect to be cured after this surgery."
    OD: Wringing hands.
    Normal Value: _____

3. **Client Value:**
    SD: "My mother and grandmother died of breast cancer..."
    OD: Carcinoma left breast, Stage 1
    Normal Value: _____

4. Client Value:

SD: "My last physical was 2 months ago."

OD: Chart reflects yearly physical 1986-1991.

Normal Value: _____

_____

•Division #13: Ventilation SD: p. 32, OD: p. 42

1. Client Value:

SD: "I wheeze when I get asthma."

OD: Minimal wheezing upon expiration.

Normal Value: _____

_____

2. Client Value:

SD: "I never smoke."

OD: Chest x-ray negative

Normal Value: _____

_____

4. Client Value:

SD: "My eyes and nose have been itching."

OD: Nasal turbinates pale and edematous; lacrimation

Normal Value: _____

_____

3. **Pattern or Division Identification:** *What data are related? Under which pattern or division should the data be grouped? What patterns are dysfunctional based on abnormal values?*

A *pattern* or *division* is a composite of similar pieces of data and represents a sequence of behavior over a period of time rather than isolated incidents. Health patterns and diagnostic divisions aid in the organization of the gathered data. Similar data is clustered under a pattern or division. Information gaps are filled by reassessing the client.

A pattern or division is deemed functional if the majority of data fall within the normal range of values and standards, thus representing the client's strengths. A pattern or division is judged dysfunctional by the nurse if the clustered data fail to meet normal or standard values, representing the client's weaknesses. A dysfunctional pattern or division may or may not lead to disease.

Nursing assessment models such as Gordon's (1989) 11 Functional Health Patterns and Doenges 13 Diagnostic Divisions serve to organize the nursing history, physical examination and grouping of nursing diagnoses. The functional health patterns and diagnostic divisions assist the nurse to identify the appropriate nursing diagnosis based on the data collected during the initial assessment. All patterns and diagnostic divisions are assessed. In case study #1, similar data were clustered under Gordon's Functional Health Patterns. In case study #2, similar data were clustered under Doenges and Moorhouse's Diagnostic Divisions. See Appendix A, p. 133-136 for a listing of clustered subjective and objective data related to Gordon's patterns. See Appendix B, p. 137-139 for a listing of clustered subjective and objective data related to Doenges and Moorhouse's Diagnostic Divisions.

The following examples illustrate a dysfunctional health pattern and a diagnostic division as the clustered data was not within normal limits.

Example of Dysfunctional Nutritional-Metabolic Pattern (Gordon's Patterns Listed in Appendix A, p. 133-136)

Subjective Data	Objective Data	Normal value
"I feel nauseated."	Vomited 100cc	No vomiting
"My skin feels dry."	Skin turgor: skin returned 10 sec	Skin returns immediately
"I am thirsty."	24 hour Intake 1000 Output 2000	24 hour Intake 2500 Output 2500

Example of Dysfunctional Diagnostic Division: Activity/Rest (Doenges and Moorhouse's Divisions Listed in Appendix B, p. 137-139)

Subjective Data	Objective Data	Normal Value
"My heart is pounding"	Pulse 100 bounding	70 male 75 female
"My blood pressure is high."	BP 180/90 lying	BP 120/80 Age 50
"My feet are swollen."	2+ edema	No edema

Exercise G: Identification of Dysfunctional Health Patterns

The purpose of Exercise G is to utilize critical thinking to identify dysfunctional health patterns in case study #1. Subjective and objective data were compared to normal values in Exercise E, p. 45-51. Based on your findings in Exercise E, identify the dysfunctional patterns that is, patterns demonstrating the majority of abnormal values and standards. Mark (X) by YES or NO. YES means the pattern was dysfunctional. NO means the pattern was not dysfunctional. Write rationale to support your judgement for answering YES or NO. Rationale is the logical or fundamental reason for the selection of your response. An example has been cited for Pattern #1: Health Perception-Health Management.

•Pattern #1: Health Perception-Health Management p. 45
Dysfunctional: YES X   NO __
Rationale: Subjective data (e.g.,increase in joint pain) and objective data(e.g.,elevatedWBC)
manifested the signs and symptoms of inflammation and infection, resulting in
an exacerbation of the rheumatoid arthritis joint pain.

•Pattern #2: Nutritional-Metabolic p. 46
Dysfunctional: YES ___   NO __
Rationale: _____
_____
_____

•Pattern #3: Elimination p. 46
Dysfunctional: YES ___   NO __
Rationale: _____
_____
_____

•Pattern #4: Activity-Exercise p. 47
Dysfunctional: YES ___   NO __
Rationale: _____
_____
_____

•Pattern #5: Sleep-Rest p. 48
Dysfunctional: YES ___   NO __
Rationale: _____
_____
_____

•Pattern #6: Cognitive-Perceptual p. 48
Dysfunctional: YES ___   NO __
Rationale: _____
_____
_____

•Pattern #7: Self-Perception/Self-Concept   p. 49
Dysfunctional:I YES ___   NO __
Rationale: _____
_____
_____

•Pattern #8:   Role-Relationship   p. 49
Dysfunctional: YES ___   NO __
Rationale: _____
_____
_____

•Pattern #9:   Sexuality-Reproductive   p. 50
Dysfunctional: YES ___   NO __
Rationale: _____
_____
_____

•Pattern #10:   Coping-Stress Tolerance   p. 50
Dysfunctional: YES ___   NO __
Rationale: _____
_____
_____

•Pattern #11:   Value-Belief   p. 51
Dysfunctional: YES ___   NO __
Rationale: _____
_____
_____

Exercise H: Identification of Dysfunctional Diagnostic Divisions

The purpose of Exercise H is to utilize critical thinking to identify dysfunctional diagnostic divisions in case study #2. Subjective and objective data were compared to normal values in Exercise F, p. 53-59. Based on the findings in Exercise F, identify the divisions that were dysfunctional, that is, the divisions demonstrating a majority of abnormal values and standards. Mark (X) by YES or NO. YES means the division was dysfunctional. NO means the division was not dysfunctional. Write rationale to support your judgement for answering YES or NO. Rationale is the logical or fundamental reason for the selection of your response. An example has been cited for diagnostic division #1: Activity-Rest.

•**Division #1: Activity-Rest p. 53**
Dysfunctional: YES x   NO __
Rationale: Slept 2-3 hours per night past 2 months. Change in sleep habit from optimal adult
sleep pattern of 7-8 hours for age. Subjective data (e.g., verbal expression of
fatigue) and objective data (e.g., dark circles under eyes) reflect sleep deprivation.

•**Division #2: Circulation p. 54**
Dysfunctional: YES ___   NO __
Rationale: _____
_____
_____

•**Division #3: Elimination p. 54**
Dysfunctional: YES ___   NO __
Rationale: _____
_____
_____

•**Division #4: Emotional Reactions p. 54**
Dysfunctional: YES ___   NO __
Rationale: _____
_____
_____

•**Division #5: Food-Fluid p. 55**
Dysfunctional: YES ___   NO __
Rationale: _____
_____
_____

•**Division #6: Hygiene p. 56**
Dysfunctional: YES ___   NO __
Rationale: _____
_____
_____

•Division #7:   Neurologic   p. 56

Dysfunctional: YES ___   NO __

Rationale: _____

_____

_____

•Division #8:   Pain   p. 56

Dysfunctional: YES ___   NO __

Rationale: _____

_____

_____

•Division #9:   Relationship Alterations   p. 57

Dysfunctional: YES ___   NO __

Rationale: _____

_____

_____

•Division #10:   Safety   p. 58

Dysfunctional: YES ___   No ___

Rationale: _____

_____

_____

•Division #11:   Sexuality   p.58

Dysfunctional: YES ___   NO __

Rationale: _____

_____

_____

•Division #12:   Teaching-Learning   p. 58

Dysfunctional: YES ___   NO __

Rationale: _____

_____

_____

•Division #13:   Ventilation   p. 59

Dysfunctional: YES ___   NO __

Rationale: _____

_____

_____

Step 2: Nursing Diagnosis

PURPOSE

The nursing diagnosis step permits the nurse to analyze and synthesize the clustered data listed under the dysfunctional health patterns and diagnostic divisions. A nursing diagnosis is formulated based on the response of the client to changes in health status, problems identified, and the nurse's ability to help find a solution.

DEFINITION OF NURSING DIAGNOSIS

Nursing diagnosis is a clinical judgment about individual, family, or community responses to actual and potential health problems/life processes. Nursing diagnoses provide the basis for selection of nursing interventions to achieve outcomes for which the nurse is accountable (Approved by the membership at the North American Nursing Diagnosis Association (NANDA), Ninth Conference, March 1990).

NURSING DIAGNOSTIC STATEMENT

Nursing Diagnostic Statement describes the health status of the client and factors contributing to the status. A nursing diagnostic statement is written by the nurse for problems identified. The following components make up a three part nursing diagnostic statement.

1. Nursing Diagnosis
2. Etiology
3. Defining Characteristics

1. Nursing Diagnosis: *What changes have occurred in the client's health?*

The nursing diagnosis is a statement that describes alterations in the client's health status. Alterations cause problems and untoward changes in the client's ability to function. The nursing diagnosis is a concise phrase or term. It represents a cluster of defining characteristics that fail to meet expected normal values. The nurse identifies a nursing diagnosis on the NANDA list that reflects a change in the client's status. NANDA's 1990 list of approved nursing diagnoses, etiologies, and defining characteristics are listed in Appendix D, p. 143-156.

Nursing diagnoses provide a foundation for establishing outcome criteria for nursing care and determining the interventions required to achieve the outcomes. If the nurse encounters difficulties selecting a nursing diagnosis, information gaps may exist. The nurse reassesses the client for further data.

Examples of NANDAs Nursing Diagnoses (see Appendix D, p. 143-156, for a complete listing). NOTE: The following nursing diagnoses will be threaded throughout the remainder of the workbook in the boxed examples.
Activity Intolerance
Ineffective Airway Clearance

---

2. Etiology: *What is causing the changes in client's health status?*

The *etiology statement* reflects the cause of the client's problem that has lead to changes in the client's health status. The cause can be attributed to behaviors of the client, pathophysiological, psychosocial, situational changes in lifestyle, developmental age, cultural and environmental factors. The cause of the changes are within the realm of nursing to treat. The phrase related to (R/T) serves to connect the nursing diagnosis and etiology statements. Etiologies applicable to each nursing diagnosis are noted in the NANDA list (Appendix D, p. 143-156).

Nursing diagnoses are applicable to all areas of nursing such as medical and surgical, maternal and child health, pediatric, psychiatric, and community health. However, the etiology or cause of a problem may differ. For example, *Activity Intolerance* related to immobility, may be the diagnostic statement for an adult with a stroke, and *Activity Intolerance* related to imbalance between oxygen supply and demand, may be the diagnostic statement for an child with congenital heart disease. For example, *Ineffective Airway Clearance* related to altered level of consciousness, may be the diagnostic statement for an adult with a stroke, and *Ineffective Airway Clearance* related to decreased energy level, may be the diagnostic statement for a child with congenital heart disease.

Examples of Etiologies for Nursing Diagnoses: Activity Intolerance and Ineffective Airway Clearance based on the above examples.

Nursing Diagnosis: *Activity Intolerance*
Possible Etiologies:
1. Immobility
2. Generalized weakness
3. Imbalance between oxygen supply and demand
4. Sedentary life style
5. Bedrest

Stroke Client

The nurse selected immobility as the etiology or cause of the client's problem. Nursing Diagnosis: *Activity Intolerance related to immobility.*

Congenital Heart Client

The nurse selected imbalance between oxygen supply and demand as the cause of the client's problem. Nursing diagnosis: *Activity Intolerance related to imbalance between oxygen supply and demand.*

- -

Nursing Diagnosis: **Ineffective Airway Clearance**
Possible Etiologies:
1. Decreased energy/fatigue level
2. Altered level of consciousness
3. Obstruction
4. Tracheobronchial infection
5. Trauma
6. Excess thick secretions
7. Pain
8. Perceptual/cognitive impairment

Stroke Client

The nurse selected altered level of consciousness as the cause of the client's problem. Nursing Diagnosis: *Ineffective Airway Clearance related to altered level of consciousness.*

Congenital Heart Client

The nurses selected decreased energy level as the cause of the client's problem. Nursing Diagnosis: *Ineffective Airway Clearance related to decreased energy level.*

3. Defining Characteristics: *What signs and symptoms provide evidence to support the selection of a nursing diagnosis?*

The defining characteristics (signs and symptoms) are a cluster of clinical cues that describe the behaviors, signs and symptoms that represent a nursing diagnosis. The defining characteristics, gathered during the assessment step, provide evidence that a health problem exists. The symptoms (subjective data) are changes which the client feels and expresses verbally to the nurse. Refer to Exercise A, p. 25-28, and Exercise B, p. 29-32 on subjective data. The signs (objective data) are observable changes in the client's health status. Refer to Exercise C, p. 35-38, and Exercise D, p. 39-42 on objective data.

Use the phrase *as evidenced by* (AEB) to connect the etiology and defining characteristic statements. The defining characteristics provide sufficient evidence to support the nursing diagnosis. Avoid basing a nursing diagnosis on one piece of data. Identify a minimum of three signs and three symptoms to provide sufficient evidence to support the selection of a nursing diagnosis.

Refer to Appendix A, p. 133-136, for other examples of defining clustered characteristics based on Gordon's Functional Health Patterns. Refer to Appendix B, p. 137-139, for other examples of defining clustered characteristics based on Doenges and Moorhouse's Diagnostic Divisions. Refer to Appendix D, p. 143-156, for NANDA's list of nursing diagnoses and defining characteristics.

Examples of Defining Characteristics Based on the Examples on p. 68

Stroke Client
Nursing Diagnosis: *Activity Intolerance*
Etiology: related to immobility
Defining Characteristics: as evidenced by

Subjective Data	Objective
"I am too weak to walk."	Unable to walk 5 feet
"I feel fatigued."	Pulse 100 upon exertion
"I feel short of breath."	Respiration 28, labored

Congenital Heart Client
Nursing Diagnosis: *Activity Intolerance*
Etiology: related to imbalance between oxygen supply and demand
Defining Characteristics: as evidenced by

Subjective Data	Objective Data
"I get tired when I play."	Dyspnea and cyanosis upon exertion
"It is hard to breathe."	Hypotonia
"My legs feel weak."	

- -

Stroke Client
Nursing Diagnosis: *Ineffective Airway Clearance*
Etiology: related to altered level of consciousness
Defining Characteristics: as evidenced by

Subjective Data	Objective Data
"I feel congested."	Coughed and expectorated copious amounts
"My chest hurts when I breathe."	of tenacious greenish sputum
"I am short of breath."	Crackling sounds right lower lobe
	Respirations 26

Congenital Heart Client
Nursing Diagnosis: *Ineffective Airway Clearance*
Etiology: related to decreased energy level
Defining Characteristics: as evidenced by

Subjective Data	Objective Data
"I cannot breathe."	Respirations 30, shallow
"I feel plugged up."	Crackling right lower lobe
"I cannot cough."	Inability to cough up sputum

Actual and Potential Nursing Diagnosis

Nursing diagnoses reflect actual or potential (high risk) problems that require resolution.

An *actual nursing diagnosis* denotes a deviation from normal health status (e.g., Activity intolerance). An actual nursing diagnosis is a three part statement: (1) nursing diagnosis (2) related to (etiology) (3) as evidenced by (defining characteristics).

Examples of Three Part Nursing Diagnostic Statements Based on Examples on p. 68

Stroke Client

Activity Intolerance (**nursing diagnosis**) related to immobility (**etiology**) as evidenced by verbal expressions fatigue, inability to walk 5 feet, pulse 100 upon exertion (**defining characteristics**).

Congenital Heart Client

Activity Intolerance (**nursing diagnosis**) related to imbalance between oxygen supply and demand (**etiology**) as evidenced by dyspnea and cyanosis upon exertion; hypotonia (**defining characteristics**).

- -

Stroke Client

Ineffective Airway Clearance (**nursing diagnosis**) related to altered level of consciousness (**etiology**) as evidenced by coughed and expectorated copious amounts of greenish sputum; crackling right lower lobe (**defining characteristics**).

Congenital Heart Client

Ineffective Airway Clearance (**nursing diagnosis**) related to decreased energy level (**etiology**) as evidenced by verbal expressions, shortness of breath, crackling right lower lobe, respirations 30 and shallow (**defining characteristics**).

A *potential (high risk) nursing diagnosis* denotes the presence of risk factors that may cause (etiology) an actual health problem in the future. At the time of the nurse's initial assessment, the client had not demonstrated defining characteristics to support the formulation of an actual nursing diagnosis. Therefore, a potential nursing diagnosis is formulated. A potential nursing diagnosis is a two part statement: (1) Potential nursing diagnosis (2) related to (etiology).

Example of a Two Part Potential (High Risk) Nursing Diagnostic Statement Based on the Examples on p. 68

Stroke Client

Potential for injury (**potential nursing diagnosis**) related to immobility (**etiology**).

Congenital Heart Client

Potential for infection (**potential nursing diagnosis**) related to inadequate primary defenses (**etiology**)

Grouping of Nursing Diagnoses for Functional Health Patterns and Diagnostic Divisions

Nursing diagnoses are grouped under Gordon'sFunctional Health Patterns (Appendix E, p. 157-158), and Doenges and Moorhouse's Diagnostic Divisions (Appendix F, p. 159-160).

Exercise I: Formulating a Three Part Nursing Diagnostic Statement

The purpose of Exercise I is to learn to formulate an actual three part nursing diagnostic statement. The health patterns listed below were identified as dysfunctional in Exercise G, p. 63-64. For each dysfunctional pattern, formulate a minimum of one nursing diagnostic statement for the client in case study #1. Refer to the nursing diagnoses listed under each of Gordon's Functional Health Patterns in Appendix E, p. 157-158. Refer to NANDA list in Appendix D, p. 143-156, for definitions of nursing diagnoses to determine if you have selected the appropriate nursing diagnosis. An example of a nursing diagnosis has been cited for the dysfunctional pattern: Health Perception-Health Management.

1. Nursing Diagnostic Statement for Dysfunctional Pattern:

•Health Perception/Health Management

Nursing Diagnosis: Altered protection

Etiology (Related to): immunosuppression

Defining Characteristics (as evidenced by): warmth, redness, edema left wrist/foot; 9/1/91

WBC 11,000; bunion culture positive

staphylococcus aureus .

2. Nursing Diagnostic Statement for Dysfunctional Pattern:

•Nutritional-Metabolic

Nursing Diagnosis: _____

Etiology (Related to): _____

Defining Characteristics (as evidenced by): _____

_____

_____

3. Nursing Diagnostic Statement for Dysfunctional Pattern:

•Activity-Exercise

Nursing Diagnosis: _____

Etiology (Related to): _____

Defining Characteristics (as evidenced by): _____

_____

_____

4. Nursing Diagnostic Statement for Dysfunctional Pattern:

•Sleep-Rest

Nursing Diagnosis: _____

Etiology (Related to): _____

Defining Characteristics (as evidenced by): _____

_____

_____

5. Nursing Diagnostic Statement for Dysfunctional Pattern:

•Cognitive-Perceptual

Nursing Diagnosis: _____

Etiology (Related to): _____

Defining Characteristics (as evidenced by): _____

_____

_____

6. Nursing Diagnostic Statement for Dysfunctional Pattern:

•Self-Perception/Self-Concept

Nursing Diagnosis: _____

Etiology (Related to): _____

Defining characteristics as evidenced by: _____

_____

_____

7. Nursing Diagnostic Statement for Dysfunctional Pattern:

•Sexuality-Reproductive

Nursing Diagnosis: _____

Etiology (Related to): _____

Defining Characteristics (as evidenced by): _____

_____

_____

Exercise J: Formulating a Three Part Nursing Diagnostic Statement

The purpose of Exercise J is to learn to formulate an actual three part nursing diagnostic statement. The diagnostic divisions listed below were identified as dysfunctional in Exercise H, p. 65-66. For each diagnostic division, formulate a minimum of one nursing diagnostic statement for the client in case study #2. Refer to the nursing diagnoses listed under each of Doenges and Moorhouse's Diagnostic Divisions, in Appendix F, p. 159-160. Refer to Appendix D, p. 143-156, for definitions of nursing diagnoses to determine if you selected the appropriate nursing diagnosis. An example of a nursing diagnosis has been cited for the dysfunctional division: Activity-Rest.

1. Nursing Diagnostic Statement for Dysfunctional Division:

•Activity-Rest

Nursing Diagnosis: Sleep-pattern disturbance

Etiology (Related to): personal stress

Defining Characteristics (as evidenced by): ptosis of eyelids, dark circles under eyes, verbalized inability to sleep.

2. Nursing Diagnostic Statement for Dysfunctional Division:

•Elimination

Nursing Diagnosis: _____

Etiology (Related to): _____

Defining Characteristics (as evidenced by): _____

_____

_____

3. Nursing Diagnostic Statement for Dysfunctional Division:

•Emotional reactions

Nursing Diagnosis: _____

Etiology (Related to): _____

Defining Characteristics (as evidenced by): _____

_____

_____

4. Nursing Diagnostic Statement for Dysfunctional Division:

•Food-fluid

Nursing Diagnosis: _____

Etiology (Related to): _____

Defining Characteristics (as evidenced by): _____

_____

5. Nursing Diagnostic Statement for Dysfunctional Division:

•Pain

Nursing Diagnosis: _____

Etiology (Related to): _____

Defining Characteristics (as evidenced by): _____

_____

_____

6. Nursing Diagnostic Statement for Dysfunctional Division:

•Relationship alterations

Nursing Diagnosis: _____

Etiology (Related to): _____

Defining Characteristics (as evidenced by): _____

_____

_____

7. Nursing Diagnostic Statement for Dysfunctional Division:

•Sexuality Female

Nursing Diagnosis: _____

Etiology (Related to): _____

Defining Characteristics (as evidenced by): _____

_____

_____

8. Nursing Diagnostic Statement for Dysfunctional Division:

•Teaching-Learning

Nursing Diagnosis: _____

Etiology (Related to): _____

Defining Characteristics (as evidenced by): _____

_____

_____

9. Nursing Diagnostic Statement for Dysfunctional Division:

•Ventilation

Nursing Diagnosis: _____

Etiology (Related to): _____

Defining Characteristics (as evidenced by): _____

_____

_____

Step 3: Planning

PURPOSE

The planning step affords the nurse, client, family and significant other an opportunity to formulate a mutually agreed upon plan of action aimed at resolving the client's problems.

COMPONENTS OF THE PLANNING STEP

1. Priority Ranking of Nursing Diagnosis
2. Establishing Outcome Criteria
3. Writing Nursing Orders
4. Writing a Nursing Care Plan

1. Priority Ranking of Problems: *What is the urgency of treating each problem? Which problems should be resolved first?*

Upon assessment, the nurse encounters multiple problems presented by the client. After formulating nursing diagnoses for the problems, the nurse initiates a *priority ranking* of the nursing diagnoses. The ranking of nursing diagnoses permits the nurse, client, family and significant other to arrange the client's problems in order of their importance and urgency.

The nursing diagnoses are ranked high, medium to low priority. The nurse, client, family and significant other focus efforts on resolving the client's high priority problems first. High priority problems reflect a life threatening situation (e.g., airway clearance). Medium priority problems deal with nonemergency, nonlife threatening needs of the client (e.g., personal hygiene). Low priority problems may not be directly related to the specific illness or prognosis (e.g., financial problems). A high priority problem (e.g., establishing a clear airway), requires prompt attention before a low priority problem (e.g., meeting the client's social needs).

Priorities may change after the initial assessment of the client, causing a shift in their importance. For example, a client was initially treated for the nursing diagnosis *Activity Intolerance*. Upon reassessing the client, the nurse noted that the client complained of shortness of breath, respirations 30 and shallow, crackling sounds right lower lobe. The problem of maintaining a clear airway due to *Ineffective Airway Clearance* constituted a higher priority than *Activity Intolerance*.

Maslow's hierarchy of needs (1968) (Figure 2-2) assists the nurse in the priority ranking of nursing diagnoses. The hierarchic framework includes physiologic and psychologic needs. The five levels of the hierarchy are: (1) physiologic, (2) safety and security, (3) love and belonging, (4) self-esteem, and (5) self-actualization. Physiological needs are satisfied before higher level needs such as self-actualization. For example, a person who lacks food will search for food before seeking fulfillment of career goals.

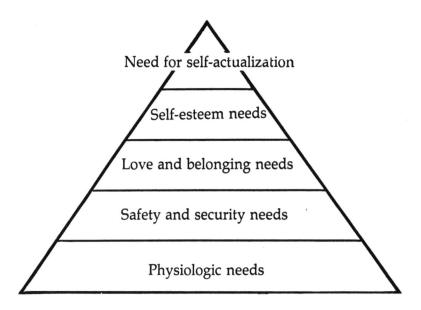

Figure 2-2: Maslow's Hierarchy of Needs

The following examples depict human needs identified on Maslow's hierarchy needs

---

Examples of Physiological Needs

Respiration	Hydration	Skin care
Circulation	Pain avoidance	Rest/Mobility
Temperature	Nutrition	Elimination

Examples of Safety and Security Needs

Environment free of hazards	Clothing
Stable living condition	Protection
Societal rules and laws	Free of infection
Free of threats real or imagined	Free of fear

Examples of Love and Belonging Needs

Affection/Sexuality
Affiliation with a group
Relationship to friends, family, peers and the community

Examples of Self-Esteem Needs

Securing the respect of colleagues
Development of feelings of competence
Feelings of self-worth and self-approval

Examples of Self-Actualization Needs

All the lower level needs have been met
Content with self and the environment

Examples of Priority Ranking of Nursing Diagnoses Using Maslow's Hierarchy of Needs Based on Examples on p. 68

Nursing Diagnoses	Maslow's Needs	Ranking
Stroke Client		
Ineffective Airway Clearance	Physiologic	High
Activity Intolerance	Physiologic	Medium
Potential for Injury	Safety/security	Medium
Congenital Heart Client		
Ineffective Airway Clearance	Physiologic	High
Activity Intolerance	Physiologic	Medium
Potential for Infection	Safety	Medium

Exercise K: Ranking Nursing Diagnoses

The purpose of Exercise K is to learn to rank nursing diagnoses in order of importance starting with #1 as the highest priority (life threatening) to the lowest priority (self-actualization). Rank the nursing diagnoses identified in Exercise I, p. 71-72, case study #1, in order of high, medium to low priority. An example has been provided based on Exercise I.

Nursing Diagnoses	Maslow's Needs	Ranking
1. Altered Protection	Physiological	High
2.		
3.		
4.		
5.		
6.		
7.		

Exercise L: Ranking Nursing Diagnoses

The purpose of Exercise L is to learn to rank nursing diagnoses in order of importance starting with #1 as the highest priority (life threatening) to the lowest priority (self-actualization). Rank the nursing diagnoses identified in Exercise J, p. 73-75, case study #2, in order of high, medium to low priority. An example has been provided based on Exercise J.

Nursing Diagnoses	Maslow's Needs	Ranking
1. Ineffective airway clearance	Physiological	High
2.		
3.		
4.		
5.		
6.		
7.		
8.		
9.		

2. Establishing Outcome Criteria: *What end results measure resolution of the client's problems?*

Outcome criteria are the realistic, measurable goals and objectives the client is expected to achieve. Outcome criteria represent the yardsticks for measuring the end results of nursing care. Outcome criteria are the aim toward which healthcare is directed and the basis for the nursing care plan.

Outcome criteria are consistent with therapies of the multidisciplinary team. For example, outcome criteria mesh with the outcomes set by the dietitian, physical and occupational therapists, physician, social worker and others. Outcome criteria are mutually set with the client, family and significant others. Failure of the client and significant others to agree with the identified outcomes, and the identification of unrealistic outcomes impedes resolution of the problem.

Goals, objectives, expected outcomes and desired client outcomes are synonyms imparting the same meaning as outcome criteria.

Outcome criteria are based on the nursing diagnosis. To formulate an outcome criterion, the nursing diagnosis is reviewed and a positive statement written to resolve the problem identified. The positive statement represents resolution or improvement of the problem.

Outcome criteria identify the steps the client must accomplish in order to achieve the outcome criteria. Outcome criteria give direction to nursing interventions and provide the foundation for evaluation of nursing care.

Each outcome criterion includes a measurable verb to facilitate the evaluation process. Measurable verbs denote actions that can be seen, heard or felt by the nurse. Outcome criteria are written on the nursing care plan. In step 5, the last step of the nursing process, the nurse returns to the written outcome criteria to evaluate whether the client has successfully fulfilled the outcomes.

COMPONENTS OF OUTCOME CRITERIA STATEMENTS

1. Subject
2. Measurable Verb
3. Outcome
4. Criteria
5. Target Time

1. *Subject* signals who is to achieve the outcome criteria. For example, the client, family, significant others and community.

Example of *Subjects* are Based on the Examples on p. 68

Stroke Client

Nursing Diagnosis: Activity Intolerance
1. *Daughter* will describe plan for client's care at home realistically by 9/30.
2. *Family friend* will walk client 50 feet every evening by 9/30.

Congenital Heart Client

Nursing Diagnosis: Ineffective Airway Clearance
1. *Client* will expectorate lung secretions unassisted by 9/20.
2. *Mother* will demonstrate use of oxygen equipment accurately by 9/30.

2. *Measurable verbs* indicate the actions, behaviors and responses of the client that can be seen, heard, smelled or felt and therefore, measurable. Write measurable verbs in the future tense by prefacing the measurable verb with the transitive verb, will. For a List of Verbs, refer to Appendix G, p. 161.

Examples of *Measurable Verbs* Based on the Examples on p. 68

Stroke Client

Nursing Diagnosis: Activity Intolerance
1. Daughter *will describe* plan for client's care at home realistically by 9/30
2. Family friend *will walk* client 50 feet every evening by 9/30.

Congenital Heart Client

Nursing Diagnosis: Ineffective Airway Clearance
1. Client *will expectorate* lung secretions unassisted by 9/20.
2. Mother *will demonstrate* use of oxygen equipment accurately by 9/30.

---

3. *Outcomes* indicate the expected physiological, psychological and life style responses of the client to the interventions. The client is expected to respond in a specific manner to a particular nursing intervention.

Examples of *Outcomes* Based on the Examples on p. 68

Stroke Client

Nursing Diagnosis: Activity Intolerance
1. Daughter will describe *plan for client care at home* realistically by 9/30.
2. Family friend will walk client *50 feet* every evening by 9/30.

Congenital Heart Client

Nursing Diagnosis: Ineffective Airway Clearance
1. Client will expectorate *lung secretions* unassisted by 9/20.
2. Mother will demonstrate *use of oxygen equipment* accurately by 9/30.

---

4. *Criteria* gauge the client's progress in achieving the outcomes. The criteria indicate the degree of proficiency required to accomplish the end results. For a list of criteria, refer to Appendix G, p. 161.

Examples of *Criteria* Based on the Examples on p. 68

Stroke Client

 Nursing Diagnosis: Activity Intolerance
1. Daughter will describe plan for client care at home *realistically* by 9/30.
2. Family friend will walk client 50 feet *every evening* by 9/30.

Congenital Heart Client

Nursing Diagnosis: Ineffective Airway Clearance
1. Client will expectorate lung secretions *unassisted* by 9/20.
2. Mother will demonstrate use of oxygen equipment *accurately* by 9/30.

---

5. *Target time* indicates the specific time period desired to achieve the outcome criteria. A time limit assists the nurse in the evaluation step to ascertain if the outcome criteria were achieved within the specified time period.

Examples of *Target Time* Based on the Examples on p. 68

<u>Stroke Client</u>

Nursing Diagnosis: Activity Intolerance
1. Daughter will describe plan for client care at home realistically *by 9/30.*
2. Family friend will walk client 50 feet every evening *by 9/30.*

<u>Congenital Heart Client</u>

Nursing Diagnosis: Ineffective Airway Clearance
1. Client will expectorate lung secretions unassisted *by 9/20.*
2. Mother will demonstrate use of oxygen equipment accurately *by 9/30.*

Examples of *Outcome Criteria Statements* Based on the Examples on p. 68

<u>Stroke Client</u>

Client (*subject*) will employ (*measurable verb*) safety measures (*outcome*) willingly (*criteria*) within 2 days (*target time*).

<u>Congenital Heart Client</u>

Mother (*subject*) will monitor (*measurable verb*) client's activity level (*outcome*) daily (*criteria*) by 9/25 (*target time*).

Exercise M: Formulating Outcome Criteria

The purpose of Exercise M is to formulate outcome criteria for case study #1. Write outcome criteria for the four nursing diagnoses with the highest priority as identified in Exercise K, p. 81. An example has been cited for case study #1.

1. Nursing Diagnosis: Altered Protection

•Outcome criteria

Subject: Client and/or wife

MeasurAble Verb: will demonstrate

Outcome: changing of dressing on left bunion

Criteria: accurately

Target Time: by 9/20/91

2. Nursing Diagnosis: _____

•Outcome Criteria

Subject: _____

Measurable Verb: _____

Outcome: _____

Criteria: _____

Target Time: _____

3. Nursing Diagnosis: _____

•Outcome Criteria

Subject: _____

Measurable Verb: _____

Outcome: _____

Criteria: _____

Target Time: _____

4. Nursing Diagnosis: _____

•Outcome Criteria

Subject: _____

_____

Measurable Verb: _____

_____

Outcome: _____

_____

Criteria: _____

_____

Target Time: _____

_____

Exercise N: Formulating Outcome Criteria

The purpose of Exercise N is to formulate outcome criteria for case study #2. Write outcome criteria for the four nursing diagnoses with the highest priority as identified in Exercise L, p. 82. An example from case study #2 has been cited.

1. Nursing Diagnosis: Ineffective Airway Clearance

•Outcome Criteria

Subject: Client

Measurable Verb: will deep breath and cough

Outcome: using abdominal and accessory muscles

Criteria: 5 min every one hour while awake

Target Time: by 9/5/91

2. Nursing Diagnosis: _____

•Outcome Criteria

Subject: _____

Measurable Verb: _____

Outcome: _____

Criteria: _____

Target Time: _____

3. Nursing Diagnosis: _____

•Outcome Criteria

Subject: _____

Measurable Verb: _____

Outcome: _____

Criteria: _____

Target Time: _____

4. Nursing diagnosis: _____

•Outcome Criteria

Subject: _____

_____

Measurable Verb: _____

_____

Outcome: _____

_____

Criteria: _____

_____

Target Time: _____

_____

3. Writing Nursing Orders: *What actions are implemented by the nurse to assist the client in achieving the outcome criteria?*

Nursing orders are specific actions the nurse implements to assist the client in achieving outcome criteria. Nursing orders denote specific, measurable, observable, and realistic actions performed by the nurse. Nursing orders, nursing actions and nursing interventions are used interchangeably.

Nursing orders are designed to reduce or resolve the etiology (cause) of the problem described in the nursing diagnosis. Refer to NANDA's List of Approved Nursing Diagnoses (Appendix D, p. 143-156) for etiologies. Nurses caring for a client follow the nursing orders written on the nursing care plan.

COMPONENTS OF THE NURSING ORDERS ON A CARE PLAN

Date: The day, month and year is written on the nursing care plan by the nurse.
Measurable Verb: Denotes the nurses' actions that can be seen, felt and heard. For examples of measurable verbs, see List of Verbs in Appendix G, p. 161.
Subject: Reflects who will receive the nurses actions. For example, the client, the family or the community. Refer to p. 83.
Outcome: Indicates the intended end result of the nurses actions. Refer to p. 84.
Target Time: Indicates the period the nurse is to implement the nursing order. Refer to p. 85.
Nurse's Signature: Verifies the nursing order.

TYPES OF NURSING ORDERS

1. Diagnostic
2. Therapeutic
3. Teaching
4. Referral

1. *Diagnostic orders* assess the progress of the client toward achieving the stated outcome criteria by direct monitoring of the client's activities. Diagnostic orders may be used to gather additional information in order to fill information gaps.

Examples of *Diagnostic Orders* Based on the Examples on p. 68

Stroke Client

9/3/91 **(date)**   Assess **(measurable verb)** client's **(subject)** range of motion upper extremities **(outcome)** by 9/4 **(target time)**. Jolene Vezzetti, RN **(signature)**

Congenital Heart Client

9/3/91 **(date)**   Talk **(measurable verb)** with wife **(subject)** to identify fears regarding client's use of oxygen **(outcome)**, by 5pm today **(target time)**. Jolene Vezzetti, RN **(signature)**

---

2. *Therapeutic orders* prescribe actions by the nurse that directly alleviate, correct or prevent an exacerbation of the problem.

Examples of *Therapeutic Orders* Based on the Examples on p. 68

<u>Stroke Client</u>

9/3/91 **(date)**   Perform **(measurable verb)** client **(subject)** passive R.O.M left leg **(outcome)** 4 times day **(target time)**. Jolene Vezzetti, RN **(signature)**.

<u>Congenital Heart Client</u>

9/3/91 **(date)**   Suction **(measurable)** client's **(subject)** lung secretions **(outcome)** as needed **(target time)**. Jolene Vezzetti, RN **(signature)**.

---

3. *Teaching orders* promote self-care of the client by assisting the individual to acquire new behaviors that facilitate resolution of the problem. Teaching orders emphasize the active participation of the client in the responsibility for self-care. Teaching orders help prepare the client and family for discharge from the healthcare system and continued care in the home.

Examples of *Teaching Orders* Based on the Examples on p. 68

<u>Stroke Client</u>

9/3/91 **(date)**   Teach **(measurable verb)** client **(subject)** use of walker **(outcome)** by 9/8 **(target time)**. Jolene Vezzetti, RN **(signature)**.

<u>Congenital Heart Client</u>

9/5/91 **(date)**   Demonstrate **(measurabale verb)** to family **(subject)** tracheal suctioning **(outcome)** by next hospital visit **(target time)**. Jolene Vezzetti, RN **(signature)**

---

4. *Referral orders* emphasize the role of the nurse as coordinator and manager of client care within the healthcare team. Referral orders specify additional consultations needed within or outside the discipline of nursing.

Example of *Referral Orders* Based on the Examples on p. 68

<u>Stroke Client</u>

9/6/91 **(date)**   Consult **(measurable verb)** with James Jason, physical therapist **(subject)**, regarding client's progress with the walker **(outcome)** by 9/8 **(target time)**. Jolene Vezzetti, RN **(signature)**.

<u>Congenital Heart Client</u>

9/6/91 **(date)**   Refer **(measurable verb)** mother **(subject)** to city health department special services for children **(outcome)** by 9/10 **(target time)**. Jolene Vezzetti, RN **(signature)**

Exercise O: Writing Nursing Orders
The purpose of Exercise O is to learn to write nursing orders for outcome criteria. Using the outcome criteria listed in Exercise M, p. 87-88, case study #1, write one nursing order for each outcome criterion.

1. Outcome Criterion: Client and wife will demonstrate changing of dressing on left bunion accurately by 9/20/91

•Nursing Order

Measurable Verb: Teach

Subject: client and wife

Outcome: dressing change on bunion

Target Time: by 9/5/91

Signature: Cyndie Smith, RN

2. Outcome Criterion:

•Nursing Order

Measurable Verb:

Subject:

Outcome:

Target Time:

Signature:

3. Outcome Criterion:

•Nursing Order

Measurable Verb:

Subject:

Outcome:

Target Time:

Signature:

4. Outcome Criterion: _____

_____

_____

_____

•Nursing Order

Measurable Verb: _____

Subject: _____

Outcome: _____

Target Time: _____

Signature: _____

Exercise P: Writing Nursing Orders

The purpose of Exercise P is to learn to write nursing orders for outcome criteria. Using the outcome criteria listed in Exercise N, p. 89-90, case study #2, write one nursing order for each outcome criterion.

1. Outcome Criterion: <u>Client will deep breath and cough using abdominal and accessory</u> <u>muscles 5 minutes every one hour while awake by 9/5/91.</u>

•Nursing Order

Measurable Verb: <u>Explain and demonstrate</u>

Subject: <u>to client</u>

Outcome: <u>therapeutic effects of deep breathing/coughing 5 minutes q1h</u>

Target Time: <u>by 9/3/91</u>

Signature: <u>Kathy Mayer, RN</u>

2. Outcome Criterion: _____

_____

_____

_____

•Nursing Order

Measurable Verb: _____

Subject: _____

Outcome: _____

Target Time: _____

Signature: _____

3. Outcome Criterion: _____

_____

_____

_____

•Nursing Order

Measurable Verb: _____

Subject: _____

Outcome: _____

Target Tme: _____

Signature: _____

4. Outcome Criterion: _____

_____

_____

_____

•Nursing Order

Measurable Verb: _____

Subject: _____

Outcome: _____

Target Time: _____

Signature: _____

Writing the Nursing Care Plan

After completion of the assessment, nursing diagnosis and planning steps, the nurse writes a nursing care plan for the client's care. The nursing care plan resembles a blueprint, a carefully designed plan. The nursing care plan organizes information about the health status of the client. The nursing care plan is an individualized plan of care, customized to resolve the client's problems.

The nursing care plan is written upon the client's admission into the healthcare system. The nursing care plan may be written on a designated healthcare form or on a computer program. On the nursing care plan, write with accepted abbreviations and key phrases instead of complete sentences. Write the nursing care plan in black permanent ink.

The nursing care plan is reviewed by the nurse prior to initiating care. The registered nurse utilizes the nursing care plan to formulate assignments for other registered nurses, licensed practical nurses, nurses aides and technicians.

The nurse evaluates the client's progress toward resolution of the problems. The nursing care plan is reviewed and revised on a timely basis. The nursing care plan is a permanent part of the client's medical record.

Benefits of Nursing Care Plans
1. Aid in the delivery of quality care.
2. Increase communication, organization and evaluation of nursing care.
3. Data base for making out assignments and allocating time and resources.
4. Data base for distribution of resources in a healthcare center by administration.
5. Data base for quality assurance audits.
6. Benefits the nursing discipline by identifying nursing's unique contribution to client care.

Example of a Nursing Care Plan Based on the Example on p. 68, the Stroke Client. Functional Health Patterns are the Assessment Framework.

ASSESSMENT	NURSING DIAGNOSTIC STATEMENT	OUTCOME CRITERIA
<u>Subjective Data</u> "I am too weak to walk." "I feel fatigued." "I feel short of breath."	*Nursing Diagnosis* Activity Intolerance, p.69 Etiology (related to) immobility	1: Client will demonstrate use of walker accurately by 9/10.
<u>Objective Data</u> Unable to walk 5 ft. Pulse 100 upon exertion Respirations 28, labored	Defining Characteristics (as evidenced by) verbalizations of fatigue, inability to walk 5 ft, pulse 100 upon exertion, p. 69	2: Daughter will describe plan for home care realistically by 9/20. 3: Family friend will walk client 50 feet every evening by 9/30.
<u>**Dysfunctional Health Pattern**</u> Activity-Exercise		

NURSING ORDERS (for)	*RATIONALE (for)*

Outcome Criteria 1:
A. Date: 9/3/91
    Teach client use of walker
    by 9/8.
    Jolene Vezzetti, RN
	Nursing Order A:
	Standing and walking extend the knee and hip joints; increases independence.

Outcome Criteria 2:
B. Date: 9/3/91
    Refer daughter to visiting
    nurse by 9/10/91.
    Jolene Vezzetti, RN
	Nursing Order B:
	Mutually agreed upon goal between client, family and nurse facilitates resolution of client's problems.

Outcome Criteria 3:
C. Date: 9/5/91
    Instruct family friend of
    therapeutic effects of
    ambulation.
    Jolene Vezzetti, RN
	Nursing Order C:
	Stress of the weight-bearing on bones decreases calcium loss from bones.

Example of a Nursing Care Plan Based on the Example on p. 68, the Congenital Heart Client. Diagnostic Divisions are the Assessment Framework.

ASSESSMENT	NURSING DIAGNOSTIC STATEMENT	OUTCOME CRITERIA
Subjective Data "I cannot breathe." "I feel plugged up." "I cannot cough."	*Nursing Diagnosis* Ineffective Airway Clearance, p. 68 Etiology (related to) decreased energy level	1: Client will expectorate lung secretions unassisted by 9/20.
Objective Data Respirations 30, shallow Crackling RLL Inability to cough-up sputum	Defining Characteristics (as evidenced by) rapid shallow respirations, verbal expressions of difficulty breathing, inability to cough-up sputum, p. 69	2: Mother will demonstrate use of oxygen equipment accurately by 9/30. 3: Parents will demonstrate suctioning of child accurately by 9/10.
Dysfunctional Diagnostic Division Ventilation		

NURSING ORDERS (for)

RATIONALE (for)

Outcome Criteria 1:
A. Date: 9/3/91
   Teach client to breathe
   deeply by 9/4/91.
   Jolene Vezzetti, RN

Nursing Order A:
Voluntary coughing in conjunction with deep breathing facilitates the movement and expectoration of respiratory tract secretions.

Outcome Criteria 2:
B. Date: 9/3/91
   Explain to Mother
   therapeutic effects of
   oxygen therapy by 9/20/91.
   Jolene Vezzetti, RN

Nursing Order B:
Additional oxygen is indicated for clients who have reduced lung diffusion of oxygen through the respiratory membrane. Teaching the family the therapeutic effects of oxygen, and use of the equipment will facilitate the home care of the client.

Outcome Criteria 3:
C. Date: 9/3/91
   Demonstrate to family
   suctioning procedure
   by 9/5/91.
   Jolene Vezzetti, RN

Nursing Order C:
Family's fears and anxieties will be reduced with an explanation of procedures. Maintaining a patent airway is a high priority need.

Exercise Q: Writing a Nursing Care Plan for Case Study #1

The purpose of Exercise Q is to write a nursing care plan for case study #1, p. 7-12. Using the following format, select one high priority nursing diagnosis from Exercise K, p. 81. Based on the nursing diagnosis that you chose, include the appropriate subjective data, objective data, dysfunctional health pattern, outcome criteria, nursing diagnostic statement, etiology and defining characteristics, nursing orders and the rationale to support each nursing order. Additional outcome criteria and nursing orders may be written.

ASSESSMENT

Subjective Data
Exercise A p. 25-28

_____
_____
_____
_____

Objective Data
Exercise C p. 35-38

_____
_____
_____
_____

DYSFUNCTIONAL HEALTH PATTERN:

_____
_____
_____

NURSING DIAGNOSTIC STATEMENT

Nursing Diagnosis

_____
_____

Etiology (related to)

_____
_____

Defining Characteristics (as evidenced by)

_____
_____
_____
_____

OUTCOME CRITERIA

1: Subject: _____

_____

Measurable Verb: _____

_____

Outcome: _____

Criteria: _____

Target Time: _____

2: Subject: _____

Measurable Verb: _____

_____

Outcome: _____

Criteria: _____

Target Time: _____

RATIONALE (for)
Nursing Order A:
_____
_____
_____
_____
_____
_____

Nursing Order B:
_____
_____
_____
_____

Nursing Order C:
_____
_____
_____
_____

NURSING ORDERS (for)
Outcome Criteria 1:
A. Date: _____
Measurable Verb: _____
Subject: _____
Outcome: _____
Target Time: _____
Signature: _____

Outcome Criteria 2:
B. Date: _____
Measurable Verb: _____
Subject: _____
Outcome: _____
Target Time: _____
Signature: _____

Outcome Criteria 3:
C. Date: _____
Measurable Verb: _____
Subject: _____
Outcome: _____
Target Time: _____
signature: _____

OUTCOME CRITERIA (CONT)
3: Subject: _____
Measurable Verb: _____
Outcome: _____
Criteria: _____
Target Time: _____

Exercise R: Writing a Nursing Care Plan for Case Study #2

The purpose of Exercise R is to write a nursing care plan for case study #2, p. 13-23. Using the following format, select one high priority diagnosis from Exercise L, p. 73-75. Based on the nursing diagnosis that you chose, include the appropriate subjective data, objective data, dysfunctional diagnostic division, outcome criteria, nursing diagnostic statement, etiology and defining characteristics, nursing order, and the rationale to support each nursing. Additional outcome criteria and nursing orders may be written.

ASSESSMENT

Subjective Data
Exercise B p. 29-32

_____

_____

_____

Objective Data
Exercise D p. 39-42

_____

_____

_____

_____

DYSFUNCTIONAL DIAGNOSTIC DIVISION

_____

_____

_____

NURSING DIAGNOSTIC STATEMENT

Nursing Diagnosis

_____

_____

Etiology (related to)

_____

_____

Defining Characteristics (as evidenced by)

_____

_____

_____

_____

OUTCOME CRITERIA

1: Subject:

_____

Measurable Verb:

_____

Outcome:

_____

Criteria:

_____

Target Time:

_____

2: Subject:

_____

Measurable Verb:

_____

Outcome:

_____

Criteria:

_____

Target Time:

_____

OUTCOME CRITERIA (CONT)

3: Subject: _____

Measurable Verb: _____

Outcome: _____

Criteria: _____

Target Time: _____

NURSING ORDERS (for)

Outcome Criteria 1:

A. Date: _____

Measurable Verb: _____

Subject: _____

Outcome: _____

Target Time: _____

Signature: _____

Outcome Criteria 2:

B. Date: _____

Measurable Verb: _____

Subject: _____

Outcome: _____

Target Time: _____

Signature: _____

Outcome Criteria 3:

C. Date: _____

Measurable Verb: _____

Subject: _____

Outcome: _____

Target Time: _____

Signature: _____

RATIONALE (for)

Nursing Order A: _____

Nursing Order B: _____

Nursing Order C: _____

Step 4: Implementation

PURPOSE

During the implementation step the nurse carries out the nursing care plan. Nursing orders are implemented to help the client meet the outcome criteria.

COMPONENTS OF THE IMPLEMENTATION STEP

1. Independent Nursing Actions
2. Collaborative Nursing Actions
3. Documentation of Nursing Actions and the Client's Response to Nursing Care

1. Independent Nursing Actions: *What actions can be implemented by the nurse without a physician's order and remain within the realm of nursing?*

Independent nursing actions are performed without a physician's order. Independent nursing actions are governed by the American Nurses Association Standards of Practice (1973); state nurse practice acts; and, healthcare facility policies.

Examples of Independent Nursing Actions Based on the Examples on p. 68

<u>Stroke Client</u>
Assessment of client
Listen to client's fears and concerns
Observation of client's response to care
Report client's status to next shift
Record the client's responses to nursing care
Teach the client to roll from side to side every hour
Demonstrate procedures to the client
Delegate tasks to nursing staff to meet needs of client
Perform full range of motion
Teach quadriceps setting
Inspect pressure areas on skin
Assess activities of daily living

<u>Congenital Heart Client</u>
Assessment of client
Teach the parents suctioning
Teach the parents auscultation of lung sounds
Report suspected murmurs
Monitor client's weight
Administer small frequent meals
Observe eating patterns
Observe for signs and symptoms of respiratory tract infection
Teach the parents temperature-taking
Schedule activities to allow for maximum rest
Assist child to select activities appropriate for condition
Introduce parents to families who have similarly affected child

---

Exercise S: Identification of Independent Nursing Actions

The purpose of Exercise S is to identify independent nursing actions. Review the nursing orders listed in Exercise O, p. 93-94, for case study #1, p. 7-12. List below the nursing orders that represent independent nursing actions.

Independent Nursing Actions:

1. Teach the client to change dressing on bunion.

2. _____

3. _____

4. _____

Exercise T: Identification of Independent Nursing Actions

The purpose of Exercise T is to identify independent nursing actions. Review the nursing orders listed in Exercise P, p. 95-96, for case study #2, p. 13-19. List below the nursing orders that represent independent nursing actions.

Independent Nursing Actions:

1. Teach client relaxation techniques. _____

2. _____
_____
_____
_____
_____

3. _____
_____
_____
_____
_____

4. _____
_____
_____
_____
_____

5. _____
_____
_____
_____
_____

2. Collaborative Nursing Actions: *Collaborative Nursing Actions are implemented when the nurse works with other healthcare team members in making joint decisions aimed at resolving the client's problems.*

Examples of Collaborative Nursing Actions

<u>Stroke Client</u>
Discuss discharge planning with multidisciplinary team.
Discuss client's fears with chaplin.
Confer with physical therapy regarding ROM exercise.
Refer client to occupational therapy.
Administer pain medication as ordered by physician.

<u>Congenital Heart Client</u>
Collect specimens as ordered by physician.
Consult with visiting nurse regarding home visit.
Refer client to respiratory therapist.
Confer with physician regarding medications.
Consult with dietitian regarding diet.

3. Documentation of Nursing Actions and Client's Responses to Nursing Care

Documentation is the act of authenticating events or activities by maintaining written records. The words: documenting, recording and charting refer to the process of writing notes on the client's record. Documentation remains the vehicle for communication from one professional to another about the status of the client. The client's record provides evidence of the independent and collaborative nursing actions implemented by the nurse, the client's response to nursing actions, and changes in the client's condition. The nurses' notes are a permanent part of the client's chart.

The frequency of documentation depends on the client's condition and the therapies administered. In a hospital, nurses' notes are written at least once per shift and address nursing diagnoses noted on the nursing care plan. The Joint Commission of Accreditation of Healthcare Organizations' standards state each client will be assessed and reassessed according to healthcare facility policies (JCAHO, 1991).

Legal Aspects of Documentation

The client's medical record is a legal document. The record is admissible in court. In a malpractice suit, the nurse's notes provide evidence of the nurse's actions. A jury will review the nurse's notes, standards of practice and care to determine if the nurse functioned as a reasonable and prudent nurse. The nurse maintains confidentiality of the information in the chart. The nurse protects the charts from unauthorized readers such as visitors. The nurse's signature at the end of a nurse's note signifies accountability for the contents of the entry. Alteration of a legal document is a felony. It is unacceptable to obliterate writing on a chart through the use of white-out, erasers, ink or other materials.

Charting in Military Time or Greenwich Time

Greenwich time is a 12 hour clock. The abbreviations a.m. and p.m denote the time of day. Military time, a 24 hour clock, eliminates confusion whether a time was a.m. or p.m. In military time, a four digit number indicates the hours and minutes. The nurse checks the healthcare policies for the correct time usage.

Comparison of Military and Greenwich Time

Military Time	Civilian Time
0100	1:00 am
0200	2:00 am
0215	2:15 am
1200	12:00 pm (noon)
1300	1:00 pm
1420	2:20 pm
1800	6:00 pm
0000	12:00 am (midnight)

TYPES OF CHARTING

Healthcare systems may implement various types of charting formats: (a) assessment forms, (b) narrative nurses notes, (c) SOAP notes, (d) FOCUS notes and (e) flowsheets and graphic records. Each format denotes the subjective and objective data, the nurses actions and the client's response to the actions. Graphic records and flowsheets depict data such as the temperature, pulse respirations, blood pressure, intake and output, medications and daily nursing care.

Assessment Forms

Assessment forms clearly delineate the data necessary for collection. Assessment forms collect subjective and objective data from the client. Avoid rewriting the information documented on the assessment form in the body of the nurses' notes unless there is a need to elaborate.

Advantages

With the increased shortage of registered nurses, assessment forms expedite the collection of data in the assessment step, and the feeding of the information into the computer. Admission assessment forms, shift or home visit assessment forms may be utilized.

Disadvantages

The disadvantage of assessment forms is the tendency for nurses to assess only the information listed on the form and failure to assess other responses of the client.

Example of Part of an Admission Assessment Tool for Gordon's 11 Functional Health Patterns
Elimination Pattern
Subjective Data

Nursing History:

  Bowel Elimination Pattern: (Describe)
  Frequency?_____
  Character?_____
  Discomfort?_____
  Problem in Control?_____
  Laxatives?_____

  Urinary Elimination Pattern: (Describe)
  Frequency?_____
  Problem in Control?_____

  Excess Perspiration? _____
  Odor Problems?_____

Example of Part of an Admission Assessment Tool for Doenges and Moorhouse's Diagnostic Divisions

Diagnostic Division: Pain

Subjective Data	Objective Data
Location_____	Facial grimacing_____
Intensity (0-10)_____	Guarding affected area_____
Quality_____	Emotional response_____
Duration_____	Narrowed focus_____
Radiation_____	
Precipitating factors_____	
How relieved_____	

Narrative Charting

A description of information about the client is provided through narrative charting.

Advantages

There are many advantages to narrative charting: (a) the charting is ongoing throughout the shift, (b) events are written in order of their occurrence, (c) narrative notes contain subjective and objective data, nursing actions and the client's response to nursing actions, (d) notes are written in a concise manner using phrases, and (e) narrative notes may be interspersed between SOAP and FOCUS entries.

Disadvantages

The disadvantage of narrative charting is the difficulty encountered in finding data about a specific problem without examining all of the recorded information. For this reason, flowsheets and graphic records are helpful in measuring specific variables.

Example of a Narrative Note Based on the Example on p. 68

Stroke Client

9/3/91   Nurses note: Potential for Infection:
2200   "My arm is burning." IV running left forearm. Left forearm erythematous, edematous, warm, painful to touch. IV discontinued. Warm soaks applied. Temperature (0) 100 F. degrees. Physician notified. IV nurse notified to restart IV another site. Jolene Vezzetti, RN.

SOAP Charting

SOAP charting is employed with Problem Oriented Medical Records. Problem Oriented Medical Records (POMR) reflect the problems identified by all members of the healthcare team. The problems are listed on a problem list in front of the client's chart. During the management of the client's healthcare, the healthcare team records SOAP charting on the progress notes. The charting portrays a continuous picture of the client's progress toward resolution of the problems.

Advantages

The nurse correlates SOAP charting with the nursing diagnoses noted on the nursing care plan. The nurse records the client's progress toward resolution of the identified problems.

Disadvantages

The SOAP note fails to show the sequence of events.

Components of SOAP charting

SOAP charting consists of four parts: (1) *S*ubjective data, (2) *O*bjective data, (3) *A*nalysis of data and (4) *P*lan.

S: (Subjective):   In quotation marks, the nurse writes the exact comments of the client.

O: (Objective):   The nurse records the data that the nurse saw, heard, smelled or touched.

A: (Analysis):   What does the data mean? The nurse analyzes and interprets the subjective and objective data. Progress toward resolution of the nursing diagnoses is noted. The analysis reflects the nurse's critical thinking and clinical judgment.

P: (Plan):   Records the plan to resolve the problem noted in the subjective (S), objective (O) and analysis (A).

Example of SOAP Charting Based on the Example on p. 68

Stroke Client

9/7/91   Physicians Note: Cerebrovascular Accident (CVA)
0900   *S* : "I feel congested. My chest hurts when I take a deep breath."
        O: Crackling sounds right lower lobe. Chest x-ray reveals right lower lobe infiltration. Sputum positive for streptococcus pneumonia.
        A : Client developing pneumonia due to immobility and decreased lung expansion.
        P : Treat with IVPB antibiotics. Mike Kelly, MD

9/7/91   Nurses Note: Ineffective Airway Clearance
1000   *S* : "I am short of breath. I told the Dr. that it hurts to breathe."
        O: Respirations 26, shallow. Crackling RLL.
        A : Immobility has decreased lung expansion. Ineffective airway clearance persists.
        P : Teach client to splint chest when coughing. Provide humidifier. Increase fluid intake to 3 liters qd. Consult with Dr. regarding chest physiotherapy. Jolene Vezzetti, RN

9/7/91   Dietitians Note: Special Diet
1200   *S* : "I cannot eat now. I am too tired."
        O: Consumed 25% lunch, liquids only.
        A : Decreased energy level limits ability to eat solid food.
        P : Offer liquid blenderized diet during acute phase of pneumonia. 1500 calorie daily intake. Progress to small frequent feedings. Steve Byrum, RD

Modified SOAP Charting

Modified SOAP charting may be entered by licensed practical nurses and nursing assistants according to the healthcare facilities' policy.

Components of Modified SOAP charting

S: (Subjective): In quotation marks, record the exact comments of the client.

O: (Objective): Record the data that is seen, heard, smelled or felt. The objective data validates the subjective data.

AT: (Action):   Actions the licensed practical nurse or nursing assistant implements to resolve the problem noted in the subjective and objective data.

> **Example of a Nurse's Note by Licensed Practical Nurse Based on the Example on p. 68**
> <u>Congenital Heart Client</u>
> 9/3/91   Nurses Note
> 1300   S: "I feel dizzy."
>   O: BP 90/50. Unsteady gait. Diaphoretic.
>   AT: Assisted to bed. Charge nurse informed. Janice Barsevich, LPN

FOCUS Charting

In FOCUS charting, the nurses notes focus or concentrate on a specific problem.

Advantages
Facilitates the documentation of nursing diagnoses and compels nurses to organize their thoughts succinctly.

Disadvantage
FOCUS charting fails to show the sequence of events.

Components of FOCUS Charting

FOCUS: The FOCUS Statement is the nursing diagnosis.
DATA: The nurse records the subjective and objective data that support the nursing diagnosis.
ACTION: Action reflects the immediate or future nursing actions to resolve the problem.
RESPONSE: The nurse describes the client's response to the nursing interventions.
TEACHING: The nurse describes the teaching to assist the client in resolving the problem.

> **Example of FOCUS Charting Based on the Example on p. 68**
> <u>Stroke Client</u>
> 9/7/91   Nurses Note (FOCUS): Pain
> 1100   DATA: "My chest hurts when I breathe or cough. I rate my pain a 6." Rated pain on scale 0-10.
>   Facial grimacing. Guarding behacior. BP 140/80. Pulse 100. Respirations 26.
>   ACTION: Tylenol #3 Tabs 1 (o) given.
> 1130   RESPONSE: "I rate my pain a 3." No facial grimacing. BP 120/80. Pulse 80. Respirations 20.
>   Medication relieved pain.
>   TEACHING: Taught to inform nurse before pain rating reaches 4. Taught distraction exercises.
>   Taught to deep breathe and cough 5 min. q1h. Jolene Vezzetti, RN

Flowsheets and Graphic Records

Flowsheets and graphic records reflect the client's variables that require frequent monitoring by the nurse.

Advantages
Specific variables such as pulse, blood pressure, medications, intake and outputs are recorded accurately and quickly on a flowsheet or graphic record. A flowsheet or graphic record reduces the amount of writing by the nurse. The time parameters for flowsheets and graphic records vary from minutes to days. For example, in a critical care unit, the vital signs will be monitored frequently whereas in community health, the vital signs may be monitored once a month. Abnormal data on the flowsheets and graphic records may be elaborated in the nurses' notes with additional relevant details.

Disadvantages
Failure to elaborate on changes in client's condition as evidenced by the readings on the flowsheet or graphic record.

Computer Charting
Computers facilitate the recording of client data. Nurses receive computer codes that are considered the nurse's legal signature. The quality of care is enhanced when nurses are relieved of clerical duties and charting information is readily available. Computers may be located at the client's bedside in a medical center.

Avoid Inferences
Nurses notes transmit facts. Avoid words that convey judgmental opinions or inferences on the nurse's part. Words imparting inferences are not measurable and may convey an incorrect meaning.

Examples of Incorrect Charting Using Words Conveying Inferences and Examples of Documentation

<u>Stroke Client</u>
Inference: *Poor appetite.*
       What is considered a poor appetite? The word poor is not measurable.
Fact: *Client ate 10% breakfast food: 120cc coffee, 1 piece wheat toast.*
       The amounts are quantified and measurable. The reader of the nurses notes will know the client's exact intake for breakfast.

<u>Congenital Heart Client</u>
Inference: *Client appears restless.*
       What is considered restless?
Fact: *"I did not sleep last night. I feel uptight about my daughter's problems." Pacing floor during interview. Wringing hands. Smoked 10 cigarettes in 20 minute period.*
       The nurse's note stated the facts, the comments heard (subjective data) and behaviors observed (objective data).

Examples of Words Reflecting Inferences To Avoid Using In Documentation

ambulating well	doing well	"I think..."	restless
anxious	eating well	large	rude
apparently	emotionally unstable	fair	seems
appears	good	little	slight
assume	great	managing well	uncooperative
conclude	improving	mild withdrawal	unexplainable
combative	inadvertently	much	unfortunately
coping well	incompetent	nervous	unstable
depressed	"I feel..."	obnoxious	well
difficult	inferior	poor	
disruptive	irritable	refused to cooperate	

Guidelines to Accurate Documentation
1. Identify the client's name on the health record prior to writing the nurses notes.
2. Stamp client's name and identification number on each page in the health record
3. Write legibly. Print if your writing is not legible.
4. Write in black permanent ink.
5. All entries begin with the time and date the note is written. In the body of the note, state the date and time of the event if it differs from the entry time and date.
6. End notes with signature, first and last name, and abbreviated title (RN). Print and sign your name if your signature is not legible.
7. Organize entries to flow in logical order of events.
8. Document on a timely basis that is, as events occur.

9. Avoid writing abbreviations. A jury will not understand their meaning (SOB: shortness of breath).
10. Records are chronological. Write on consecutive lines and pages. Avoid leaving blanks in lines of writing. Draw a single line to end of the line to fill the blank space.
11. Avoid leaving blank lines between entries.
12. Use a large X to fill the rest of the blank page.
13. If a writing error occurs, draw a single line through the word, and initial above the word.
14. When correcting an error, do not obliterate the word or words.
15. Do not use white-out to correct errors on the nurses notes or other records. Do not erase errors.
16. Do not write in margins or squeeze entries between lines.
17. Recopy a damaged page of the record. Recopy exactly as written onto another page. Do not destroy the original. The original page remains part of the permanent chart. Cross reference the 2 pages. On the copy write, Recopied from page...and on the original write, Recopied on page....
18. For late entries, write the date and time the late entry is written. In the body of the nurses note, record the date and time the action occurred, the late note signature and title.
19. Document noncompliant behavior (e.g., "I will not attend group therapy today.")
20. Capital letters begin each thought. Periods complete each thought (e.g., Dyspneic upon exertion. Ate 25% breakfast food).
21. Omit the word client since the health record belongs to the client.
22. Spell words correctly (e.g., Keflin; Keflex).
23. Precise measurements (metric) ensure accuracy (e.g., Drank 200cc water).

Exercise U: Narrative Nurses's Notes

The purpose of Exercise U and Exercise V is to learn to write accurate nurse's notes. For Exercise U, write a narrative nurse's note for case study #1, p. 7-12, based on the following scenario. Refer to the example for narrative notes on p. 111.

Scenario for Exercises U and V: Cyndie Smith, RN arrives in Mr. Hill's room and the following scene ensues:

Date 9/4/91 Time 1230
Mr. Hill: "I am having pain in all my joints. They really hurt. It feels like a knife is stabbing each joint."

Nurse: "How long have you been in pain? Would you please rate your pain on a scale of 0-10 with 0 no pain and 10 excruciating pain. Is the pain throbbing or sharp? What do you take to relieve the pain at home?"

Mr. Hill: "I rate my pain an 8. I take ecotrin 32 mg, 2 Tablets 4 times a day at home. I need some Tylenol #3 for this pain."

Nurse: Observes that Mr. Hill is moaning, facial muscles taut. BP 160/80. Pulse 100.

Date 9/4/91 Time 1245

Nurse: Administers Tylenol #3 2 tablets orally to Mr.Hill. Nurse returns at 1315 to check the effectiveness of the medication.

Nurse: 1315, "How would you rate your pain now Mr. Hill?" Nurse notes no facial grimacing or moaning. BP 140/80. Pulse 80.

Mr. Hill: "I feel better. I rate my pain a 4."

Nurse: "I am going to teach you rhythmic breathing to help relieve your pain."

Narrative Nurses Note

Date: _____
Time: _____
_____
_____
_____
_____
_____
_____
_____
_____
_____
_____
_____
_____

Exercise V: FOCUS Nurses Notes

The purpose of Exercise V is to learn to write accurate nurse's notes (see scenario on p. 117). For Exercise V, write a FOCUS nurse's note for case study #1, p. 7-12, based on the following scenario. Refer to the example for FOCUS notes on p. 113.

Date: _____

Time: _____

FOCUS: _____

_____

_____

_____

DATA: _____

_____

_____

_____

ACTION: _____

_____

_____

_____

RESPONSE: _____

_____

_____

_____

TEACHING: _____

_____

_____

_____

Exercise W: Writing SOAP Nurses Notes

The purpose of Exercise W is to learn to write accurate nurse's notes. Write a nurse's note for case study #2, p. 13-19, based on the following scenario. Use SOAP charting. Refer to example for SOAP notes on p. 111.

Scenario for Exercise W: Kathy Mayer, RN arrives in Mrs. Smith's room and the following scene ensues:

Date 9/3/91 Time 1400 The following scenario occurred:

Mrs. Smith: "I am having a migraine headache. I feel nauseated. Please give me some medicine."

Nurse: "Where is your headache? How would you rate the pain on a scale on 0 to 10 with 0 no pain and 10 excruciating pain? What caused the headache to start? Is the pain throbbing or sharp."

Mrs. Smith: "I rate my pain a 7. It feels like pressure over my left eye and causes my eye to tear. I am so tense about this surgery. Aspirin does not help. I take ergotamine one tablet when my headache begins."

Nurse: Observes diaphoresis. Facial grimacing. Tearing left eye. Rubbing left fore head. Palpable neck and shoulder muscles. Lights off in room. Shades on window pulled. BP 146/80 lying. Pulse 90.

Date 9/3/91 Time 1415

Nurse: Administered Ergotamine 2mg sublingual tablet.

Date 9/3/91 Time 1500

Nurse: "How would you rate your pain now Mrs. Smith?"

Mrs. Smith: "My migraine is a little better. I rate the pain a 4. My nausea is gone."

Nurse: Observes no facial grimacing. No diaphoresis No rubbing left forehead. BP 130/70. Pulse 80. "I plan to teach you distraction techniques to use when you feel another headache beginning."

Exercise W: SOAP Nurses Notes

Date: _____

Time: _____

S (Subjective): _____

_____

_____

_____

_____

O (Objective): _____

_____

_____

_____

A (Analysis): _____

_____

_____

_____

P (Plan): _____

_____

_____

_____

Date: _____

Time: _____

S (Subjective): _____

_____

_____

_____

_____

O (Objective): _____

_____

_____

_____

A (Analysis): _____

_____

_____

_____

P (Plan): _____

_____

_____

_____

Step 5:   Evaluation

PURPOSE

The evaluation step is a comparison of observed results with projected outcome criteria established in the planning step. The client exits the nursing process cycle when the outcome criteria have been achieved. The client renters the cycle (Figure 2-3) if the outcome criteria were not met.

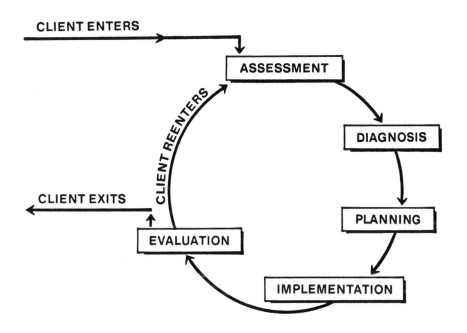

Figure 2-3: Nursing Process Cycle

COMPONENTS OF THE EVALUATION STEP

1. Achievement of Outcome Criteria
2. Effectiveness of the Steps of the Nursing Process
3. Revision or Termination of the Nursing Care Plan

1. Achievement of Outcome Criteria: *Where is the evidence to support achievement of the outcome criteria? How realistic were the outcome criteria?*

Achievement of outcome criteria by the target date is the yardstick for measurement.

Refer to p. 83-85 for an explanation of outcome criteria. The nursing care plan and nurses notes are reviewed to determine achievement of outcome criteria. The nurses' notes reflect the client's response to nursing actions and provide evidence to support the attainment of outcome criteria. When the outcome criteria are achieved, the word resolved and the date are written on the nursing care plan. If the outcome criteria were not met, the nurse reassesses the client and revises the nursing care plan.

Example of Achievement of Outcome Criteria Confirmed by Comments in Nurses Notes. Refer to Example on p. 68

<u>Stroke Client</u>

Outcome Criterion (p. 83):

9/3/91	Daughter will describe plan for client's care at home realistically by 9/30.
9/30/91	Nurse's Note: Activity Intolerance

       S: Daughter stated, "I plan to hire a nurses aide to care for my father during the day, while I am at work."

       O: Social workers note confirms nurses aide has been hired.

       A: Activity intolerance persists.

       P: Visiting nurse will teach nurses aide to perform ROM to client's extremities qid. Jolene Vezzetti, RN

- -

<u>Congenital Heart Client</u>

Outcome Criterion (p. 83):

9/3/91	Client will expectorate lung secretions unassisted by 9/20.
9/20/91	Nurse's note: Impaired airway clearance

       S: "I can cough up the stuff in my chest now."

       O: Lungs clear to auscultation.

       A: Impaired airway clearance resolved.

       P: Discontinue home visits. Clinic appointment in 3 months. Jolene Vezzetti, RN

---

2. Effectiveness of the Steps in the Nursing Process : *How accurate were the steps of the nursing process? What factors hindered achievement of the outcome criteria?*

Factors affecting the achievement of outcome criteria may occur throughout the nursing process. Factors that impede progress are: (a) information gaps occurring in the assessment, Step 1; (b) wrong nursing diagnosis identified in Step 2; (c) nursing orders not congruent with outcome criteria, Step 3; (d) failure to implement the nursing care plan, Step 4; and (e) failure to evaluate the client's progress, Step 5.

Example of Failure to Achieve Outcome Criteria Confirmed by the Nurse's Note. Refer to Example on p. 68

<u>Stroke Client</u>

Outcome Criterion (p. 83):

9/3/91	Family friend will walk client 50 feet every evening by 9/30.
9/30/91	Nurses note: Activity intolerance
1300	Family friend out of town on business for month of September. Client unable to walk 10 feet unassisted. Wife unable to walk client. Outcome criteria not met. Confer with wife and social worker regarding home care assistance by 10/1. Jolene Vezzetti, RN

- -

<u>Congenital Heart Client</u>

Outcome Criterion (p. 83):

9/3/91	Mother will demonstrate use of oxygen equipment accurately by 9/30.
9/25/91	Nurses note: Ineffective airway clearance Mother states, "I am afraid to use the oxygen tank." Nurse redemonstrated use of oxygen tank. Mother refused to return demonstration. Repeat demonstration tomorrow. Outcome criteria not met. Refer to visiting nurse upon discharge. Jolene Vezetti, RN.

---

3. Revision or Termination of the Nursing Care Plan: *Is the client ready to exit the Nursing Process Cycle? What revisions are required in the nursing care plan?*

With achievement of the outcome criteria, the client exits the nursing process cycle and the nursing care plan is terminated. The nurse writes a discharge note summarizing resolution of each nursing diagnoses. The discharge note indicates the client's status upon release from the healthcare system. Vital signs, procedures taught, medications, self-care abilities, support system and follow-up appointments are examples of information included in a discharge note.

If the outcome criteria were unmet, the client reenters the nursing process cycle. The nurse reassesses the client and revises the nursing care plan to meet current needs. A referral to another healthcare worker may be written to provide continuity of care. For example, a referral to the visiting nurse may be written requesting observation of insulin administration by the client at home.

Example of Discharge Notes Based on the Examples, p. 68

<u>Stroke Client</u>

9/30/91	Nurses Discharge Summary
1100	Nursing diagnosis: Activity intolerance
	Walked 50 feet in hallway with walker. Family friend attended physical therapy session with client 9/29. Family friend verbalized therapeutic effects ambulation. Daughter demonstrated ROM all joints correctly. Daughter identified plan for home care. Outcome criteria met.
	Jolene Vezzetti, RN

- -

<u>Congenital Heart Client</u>

9/30/91	Nurses Discharge Summary
1400	Nursing Diagnosis: Impaired airway clearance.
	Mother administered oxygen therapy correctly. Client expectorates own secretions. Lungs clear to auscultation. Outcome criteria met. Home visit by visiting nurse 10/1.
	Jolene Vezzetti, RN

Exercise X: Evaluation of Outcome Criteria

The purpose of Exercise X is to evaluate the achievement of outcome criteria noted on the nursing care plan. In Exercise M, p. 87-88, outcome criteria were identified for case study #1. Based on the scenario below, write your evaluation of whether the outcome criteria you listed in Exercise M were resolved.

Scenario as of 9/28/91: Mr. Hill is scheduled for discharge 9/30/91. Mr. Hill demonstrated the ability to walk 50 feet using a walker. The edema, redness and tenderness in his joints has subsided. His joints remain positive for subcutaneous nodules. Limited range of motion of all joints continues. Demonstrated the ability to assist with bathing, dressing and feeding self. Ate 100% of his meals. Stated, "I can taste the food now." No lesions present in his mouth. Skin turgor returns immediately. Ulcer left foot dry and culture negative. Wife demonstrated ability to change dressing on bunion using aseptic technique. Hemoglobin 14 g/dL. Hematocrit 40%. Visiting nurse to see client 10/1/91.

1. Outcome Criterion: Client and wife will demonstrate changing of dressing on bunion

accurately by 9/20.

Resolved: YES _X_   NO ____

Evaluation: Wife demonstrated changing of sterile dressing on bunion accurately. Client

unable to perform task due to limited joint mobility.

2. Outcome Criterion: _____

_____

_____

_____

_____

_____

Resolved: YES _____   NO ____

Evaluation: _____

_____

_____

_____

_____

_____

3. Outcome Criterion: _____

_____

_____

_____

_____

_____

Resolved: YES_____   NO ___
Evaluation: _____

_____

_____

_____

_____

_____

4. Outcome Criterion: _____

_____

_____

_____

_____

Resolved: YES_____   NO ___
Evaluation: _____

_____

_____

_____

_____

_____

Exercise Y: Evaluation of Outcome Criteria

The purpose of Exercise Y is to evaluate the achievement of outcome criteria noted on the nursing care plan. In Exercise N, p. 89-90 outcome criteria were identified for case study #2. Based on the scenario below, write your evaluation of whether the outcome criteria listed in Exercise N were achieved.

Scenario as of 9/13/91: Mrs. Smith had a mastectomy 9/5/91. Mrs. Smith stated that her husband was on a business trip. He did not call her until 9/6/91, two days postoperatively. Mrs. Smith's two children visited on the weekend. Mrs. Smith has cried throughout her hospitalization. Her migraine headaches persist with no relief from ergotamine. Mrs. Smith rates her anxiety level a 3 on scale 0-5. Her incision is dry and intact. No complaints of pain in incisional area on the left breast site. States she does not sleep at night. Dark circles and ptosis of eyelids present. Facial muscles taut. Verbalizes relaxation techniques. Nurse has observed client practicing guided imagery intermittently. BP 150/80 sitting. Pulse 90. Lungs clear to auscultation. No edema nasal turbinates. No nasal drainage. No tearing eyes. Priest visits Mrs. Smith daily. Continues to eat 25% of her meals. Demonstrated ability to bathe, feed and dress self. Scheduled for discharge 9/14/91.

1. Outcome Criterion: Explain and demonstrate to client therapeutic effects of deep

breathing/coughing q1h by 9/3/91.

Resolved: YES _X_ NO

Evaluation: Client observed deep breathing and coughing q1h postoperatively. Lungs clear

to auscultation. No edema nasal turbinates. No nasal drainage. R 18.

2. Outcome Criterion: _____

_____

_____

_____

_____

_____

Resolved: YES _____ NO ___

Evaluation: _____

_____

_____

_____

_____

3. Outcome Criterion: _____
_____
_____
_____
_____
_____

Resolved: YES _____   NO ___
Evaluation: _____
_____
_____
_____
_____
_____

4. Outcome Criterion: _____
_____
_____
_____
_____

Resolved: YES _____   NO ___
Evaluation: _____
_____
_____
_____
_____
_____

PART III: APPENDICES

Appendix A: Gordon's 11 Functional Health Patterns: Clustering of Subjective and Objective Data

Listed below are clustered subjective and objective data related to each functional health pattern. The list is not conclusive. In case study #1, p. 7-12, similar data were clustered under Gordon's functional health patterns.

•Pattern #1: Health Perception/Health Management

Describes the client's perception and management of health and well-being.

<u>Subjective Data</u>

Reason for admission
Prescription/nonprescription medications
Medical and social history
Expectation healthcare providers
Ongoing treatment unrelated to admission diagnosis
Clients perception of health status and well-being

<u>Objective Data</u>

General survey
Evidence of use of illicit drugs
White blood cell count
Ability to set goals; knowledge of health practices
Hygiene, grooming
Age
Occupational hazards

•Pattern #2: Nutritional/Metabolic

Describes dietary intake; fluid and electrolyte balance; condition of skin, hair and nails.

<u>Subjective Data</u>

Fat intake; Na+ intake
Appetite; caffein use
Problems with eating, swallowing, digesting
Nausea
Use alcohol
Routine hair, skin, nail, and mouth care
Allergies food
Urticaria
Weight changes
Food preferences

<u>Objective Data</u>

Prescribed diet
Percentage of food eaten
Ability swallow
Nasogastric tube
Caloric intake
Intravenous fluids
Total parenteral nutrition
Nitrogen balance
Serum albumin
Vomiting
Electrolyte values
Intake and output
Temperature
Height, weight, skin
Head, neck, hair
Nail, mouth, lips
Teeth, dentures, gums
Edema

•Pattern #3: Elimination

Describes patterns of excretory function of the bowel, bladder and skin.

<u>Subjective Data</u>

Bladder
Frequency, nocturia
Usual characteristics urine output
Problem urinating
Fluid intake pattern
Urinary tract infections

<u>Objective Data</u>

Bladder
Urine amount, color, odor
Specific gravity
Catheter, condom, ostomy
Palpable bladder
Palpable kidneys
Skin excoriation
Intake and output

Bowel
Frequency and usual characteristics of stool
Use of laxatives
Problems with constipation or diarrhea
Use stool softeners

Bowel
Stool amount, color, consistency
Abdomen soft, tender distended
Bowel sounds
Fistulas, ostomy
Drainage tubes
Skin excoriation
Roughage in diet

Skin
Excess perspiration
Odor problems

Skin
Diaphoresis
Body odor
Drainage tubes

•Pattern #4: Activity/Exercise
Describes pattern of exercise and activity, respiratory and circulatory function.

Subjective Data

Objective Data

Breathing
Shortness of breath (SOB) or pain with exercise
Smoking
History asthma, bronchitis or emphysema
Family history lung disease
Occupational hazards

Breathing
Respiratory rate, depth, rhythm
Breath sounds
Anteroposterior diameter (A-P)
Chest tubes
Presence of cough
Use accessory muscles

Circulation
Family history of heart disease
Previous myocardial infarction,
  cerebrovascular accident
Pacemaker
Intermittent claudication
Medications

Circulation
Apical rate, rhythm
Blood pressure
Peripheral pulses
Capillary refill
Skin color
Lower extremity temperature and hair loss
Blood loss/transfusions
Central venous pressure (CVP)
Clotting factors
Transaminase (SGOT)
Lactic dehydrogenase (LDH)
Creatinine phosphokinase (CPK)

Mobility
Usual exercise pattern
Leisure activities
Stair climbing
Use of cane, walker
Limitation in activities of daily living (ADL)
Gait problems
Sufficient energy to perform activities
Activities since illness

Mobility
Range of motion (ROM)
Strength, posture,
Hand grip,reflexes
Ability perform ADL:
  feeding, bathing, toileting, bed, mobility,
  dressing, shopping
Absence body part
Prosthesis
Gait, balance

•Pattern #5: Sleep/Rest
Describes patterns of sleep, rest and perception of energy level.

Subjective Data

Objective Data

Usual hours of sleep
Rested for daily activities
Complains drowsiness
Complains fatigue
Bedtime routine

Observe sleep/nap time; frequent yawning
Hypnotics, sedatives
Dark circles under eyes; ptosis eyelids
Attention span

•Pattern #6: Cognitive/Perceptual

Describes patterns of hearing, vision, taste, touch, smell, pain perception, language, memory and decision making.

Subjective Data	Objective Data
Sensory and perceptual problems: hearing, vision, touch, smell, taste	Ability to see, hear, smell, feel
	Seizure activity
English as a second language	Language spoken
Educational level	Ability to follow
Pain perception and pain management	Decision-making ability
Memory changes	Level consciousness
Rates pain on scale 0-10	Neurological exam
Use of hearing aid or glasses	Oriented to time, place, person
Recent loss of body part or function	Demonstrates accurate awareness body parts

•Pattern #7: Self Perception/Self-Concept

Describes attitudes about self and perception of abilities.

Subjective Data	Objective Data
Attitudes about self	Body posture
Impact of illness on self	Eye contact
Desire to change self	Assertive or passive: rate 1-5
Nervous or relaxed: rate 1-5	Nonverbal cues to altered self-esteem
Perceived powerlessness	Facial expressions

•Pattern #8: Role/Relationship

Describes effectiveness of roles and relationships with significant others.

Subjective Data	Objective Data
Employment	Observed interaction
Effectiveness of relationships with significant other	Passive or aggressive behavior toward others
Effect of role change on relationships	
Financial concerns	
Residence; homeless	

•Pattern #9: Sexuality/Reproductive

Describes actual or perceived satisfaction or problems with sexuality.

Subjective Data	Objective Data
Impact illness on sexuality	Breast exam
Menstrual history; children	Testicular exam
Self-breast exam	Genitalia exam
Pruritus	Lesions
Birth control measures	Drainage
History sexually transmitted disease	Venereal Disease Research Laboratory (VDRL)
	Human immunodeficiency virus (HIV)

•Pattern #10: Coping/Stress Tolerance

Describes ability to manage stress and use of support systems.

Subjective data	Objective Data
Stressors in past year	Interactions with significant others
Usual coping methods	Kinetic movements
Support system	Pacing
Use alcohol, illicit and prescribed drugs to alleviate stress	No eye contact
	Crying, voice
Effect illness on stress level	Voice tone
Rates anxiety scale 0-5	Expression

•Pattern #11: Value/Belief

Describes spirituality, values, and belief system.

<u>Subjective Data</u>

Religion; spirituality
Religious, cultural beliefs and practices;
  shared by others
Attitude toward do not resuscitate order (DNR)

<u>Objective Data</u>

Seeks spiritual assistance
Evidence of practice of values, beliefs

Adapted from: Gordon, M (1989). <u>Manual of Nursing Diagnosis.</u> New York. McGraw-Hill.

Appendix B: Doenges and Moorhouse's 13 Diagnostic Divisions: Clustering of Subjective and Objective Data

Subjective and objective data can be clustered related to each diagnostic division. In case study #2, p. 13-19, clustered data is organized by Doenges and Moorhouse's Diagnostic Divisions.

•**Diagnostic Division #1: Activity/Rest**

Describes exercise and sleep habits, and the cardiopulmonary response activity.

<u>Subjective Data</u>   <u>Objective Data</u>

•**Diagnostic Division #2: Circulation**

Describes history and present assessment of the circulatory functions.

<u>Subjective Data</u>   <u>Objective Data</u>

•**Diagnostic Division #3: Elimination**

Describes bowel and bladder functions.

<u>Subjective Data</u>   <u>Objective Data</u>

•**Diagnostic Division #4: Emotional Reactions**

Describes client's feelings of self- esteem, and emotional status.

<u>Subjective Data</u>   <u>Objective Data</u>

•Diagnostic Division #5: Food and Fluid

Describes daily dietary intake; fluid and electrolyte blance.

<u>Subjective Data</u>   <u>Objective Data</u>

•Diagnostic Division #6: Hygiene

Describes ability to perform self-care.

<u>Subjective Data</u>   <u>Objective Data</u>

•Diagnostic Division #7: Neurologic

Describes status of sensory organs and mental status.

<u>Subjective Data</u>   <u>Objective Data</u>

•Diagnostic Division #8: Pain

Describes client's perception of pain.

<u>Subjective Data</u>   <u>Objective Data</u>

•Diagnostic Division #9: Relationship Alterations

Describes support system.

<u>Subjective Data</u>   <u>Objective Data</u>

•**Diagnostic Division #10:Safety**

Describes client's allergies, and evidence of injury.

<u>Subjective Data</u>   <u>Objective Data</u>

•**Diagnostic Division #11:Sexuality**

Describes history of sexual development, and sexual concerns.

<u>Subjective Data</u>   <u>Objective Data</u>

•**Diagnostic Division #12:Teaching/Learning**

Describes the client's ability to explain and implement information.

<u>Subjective Data</u>   <u>Objective Data</u>

•**Diagnostic Division #13:Ventilation**

Describes client's ability to maintain airway clearance.

<u>Subjective Data</u>   <u>Objective Data</u>

Modified from: Doenges, M., and Moorhouse, M. (1988). <u>Nurses Pocket Guide: Nursing Diagnoses with Interventions</u>. 2nd Edition. Philadelphia, Davis.

Appendix C: NANDA TAXONOMY I REVISED-1990

•Pattern 1: Exchanging

1.1.2.1.	Altered nutrition: more than body requirements
1.1.2.2.	Altered nutrition: less than body requirements
1.1.2.3.	Altered nutrition: potential for more than body requirements
1.2.1.1.	Potential for infection
1.2.2.1.	Potential altered body temperature
1.2.2.2.	Hypothermia
1.2.2.3.	Hyperthermia
1.2.2.4.	Ineffective thermoregulation
1.2.3.1.	Dysreflexia
1.3.1.1.	Constipation
1.3.1.1.1.	Perceived constipation
1.3.1.1.2.	Colonic constipation
1.3.1.2.	Diarrhea
1.3.1.3.	Bowel incontinence
1.3.2.	Altered urinary elimination
1.3.2.1.1.	Stress incontinence
1.3.2.1.2.	Reflex incontinence
1.3.2.1.3.	Urge incontinence
1.3.2.1.4.	Functional incontinence
1.3.2.1.5.	Total incontinence
1.3.2.2.	Urinary retention
1.4.1.1.	Altered (specify type) tissue perfusion (Renal, cerebral, cardiopulmonary, gastrointestinal, peripheral)
1.4.1.2.1.	Fluid volume excess
1.4.1.2.2.1.	Fluid volume deficit
1.4.1.2.2.2.	Potential fluid volume deficit
1.4.2.1.	Decreased cardiac output
1.5.1.1.	Impaired gas exchange
1.5.1.2.	Ineffective airway clearance
1.5.1.3.	Ineffective breathing pattern
1.6.1.	Potential for injury
1.6.1.1.	Potential for suffocation
1.6.1.2.	Potential for poisoning
1.6.1.3.	Potential for trauma
1.6.1.4.	Potential for aspiration
1.6.1.5.	Potential for disuse syndrome 1
1.6.2.	Altered protection
1.6.2.1.	Impaired tissue integrity
1.6.2.1.1.	Altered oral mucous membrane
1.6.2.1.2.1.	Impaired skin integrity

•Pattern 2: Communicating

2.1.1.1.	Impaired verbal communication

•Pattern 3: Feeling

3.1.1.	Impaired social interaction
3.1.2.	Social isolation
3.2.1.	Altered role performance
3.2.1.1.1.	Altered parenting
3.2.1.1.2.	Potential altered parenting
3.2.1.2.1.	Sexual dysfunction
3.2.2.	Altered family processes
3.2.3.1.	Parental role conflict
3.3.	Altered sexuality patterns

•Pattern 4: Valuing

4.1.1.	Spiritual distress (distress of the human spirit)

•Pattern 5: Choosing

5.1.1.1.	Ineffective individual coping
5.1.1.1.1.	Impaired adjustment
5.1.1.1.2.	Defensive coping
5.1.1.1.3.	Ineffective denial
5.1.2.1.1.	Ineffective family coping: disabling
5.1.2.1.2.	Ineffective family coping: compromised
5.1.2.2.	Family coping: potential for growth
5.2.1.1.	Noncompliance (specify)
5.3.1.1.	Decisional conflict (specify)
5.4.	Health seeking behaviors (specify)

•Pattern 6: **Moving**

6.1.1.1.	Impaired physical mobility
6.1.1.2.	Activity intolerance
6.1.1.2.1.	Fatigue
6.1.1.3.	Potential activity intolerance
6.2.1.	Sleep pattern disturbance
6.3.1.1.	Diversional activity deficit
6.4.1.1.	Impaired home maintenance management
6.4.2.	Altered health maintenance

6.5.1.	Feeding self-care deficit
6.5.1.1	Impaired swallowing
6.5.1.2.	Ineffective breastfeeding
6.5.1.3.	Effective breastfeeding
6.5.2.	Bathing/hygiene self-care deficit
6.5.3.	Dressing/grooming self-care deficit
6.5.4.	Toileting self-care deficit
6.6.	Altered growth and development

•Pattern 7: **Perceiving**

7.1.1.	Body image disturbance
7.1.2.	Self-esteem disturbance
7.1.2.1.	Chronic low self-esteem
7.1.2.2.	Situational low self-esteem
7.1.3.	Personal identity disturbance

7.2.	Sensory/perceptual alterations (specify: visual, auditory, kinesthetic, gustatory, tactile, olfactory)
7.2.1.1.	Unilateral neglect
7.3.1.	Hopelessness
7.3.2.	Powerlessness

•Pattern 8: **Knowing**

8.1.1.	Knowledge deficit (specify)
8.3.	Altered thought processes

•Pattern 9: **Feeling**

9.1.1.	Pain
9.1.1.1.	Chronic pain
9.2.1.1.	Dysfunctional grieving
9.2.1.2.	Anticipatory grieving
9.2.2.	Potential for violence: self-directed or directed at others
9.2.3.	Post-trauma response

9.2.3.1.	Rape-trauma syndrome
9.2.3.1.1.	Rape-trauma syndrome: compound reaction
9.2.3.1.2.	Rape-trauma syndrome: silent reaction
9.3.1.	Anxiety
9.3.2.	Fear

Used with permission from: North American Nursing Diagnosis Association. (1990). Taxonomy I-Revised 1990. St. Louis: NANDA.

Appendix D : NANDA'S 1990 List of Approved Nursing Diagnoses, Definitions, Etiologies and Defining Characteristics

The following list of nursing diagnoses is based on NANDA'S TAXONOMY I-REVISED (1990). The list is not conclusive and requires continual research. [Brackets] indicate material added by the author.

•Activity Intolerance

Definition: A state in which an individual has insufficient physiological or psychological energy to endure or complete required or desired daily activities.

Etiology/related to factors: Bedrest; immobility; generalized weakness; sedentary life-style; imbalance between oxygen supply and demand.

Defining characteristics: Verbal report of fatigue or weakness; abnormal heart rate or blood pressure response to activity, exertional discomfort or dyspnea; electrocardiographic changes reflecting arrhythmias or ischemia.

•Altered Family Processes

Definition: The state in which a family that normally functions effectively experiences a dysfunction.

Etiology/related to factors: Situation transition; developmental crisis.

Defining characteristics: Family system unable to meet physical and emotional needs of its members; family unable to adapt to traumatic experience constructively.

•Altered Growth and Development

Definition: An individual demonstrates deviations in norms from his/her age group.

Etiology/related to factors: Inadequate caretaking; indifference, inconsistent responsiveness, multiple caretakers; separation from significant others; environmental and stimulation deficiencies; effects of physical disability; prescribed dependence.

Defining characteristics: Delay of difficulty in performing skills typical of age group; altered physical growth; inability to perform self-care or activities for age.

•Altered Health Maintenance

Definition: Inability to identify, manage, and/or seek out help to maintain health.

Etiology/related to factors: Lack of, or significant alteration in communication skills; lack of ability to make deliberate and thoughtful judgments; perceptual or cognitive impairment; lack of material resources.

Defining characteristics: Demonstrated lack of knowledge regarding basic health practices; demonstrated lack of adaptive behaviors to internal or external environmental changes; observed lack of equipment and finances.

•Altered Nutrition: Less Than Body Requirements

Definition: An individual experiences an intake of nutrients insufficient to meet metabolic needs.

Etiology/related to factors: Inability to ingest or digest food or absorb nutrients due to biological, psychological, or economic factors.

Defining characteristics: Body weight 20% or more below ideal for height and frame; reported food intake less than recommended daily allowance (RDA); reported weakness of muscles required for swallowing or mastication; inflamed buccal cavity.

•Altered Nutrition: More Than Body Requirements

Definition: An individual experiences an intake of nutrients which exceeds metabolic needs.

Etiology/related to factors: Excessive intake in relation to metabolic need.

Defining characteristics: Weight 20% over ideal for height and frame; triceps skin fold greater than 15 mm in men, 25 mm in women; observed or reported sedentary activity level.

•Altered Nutrition: Potential for More Than Body Requirements

<u>Definition</u>: An individual is at risk for experiencing an intake of nutrients which exceeds metabolic needs.
<u>Related to the presence of risk factors</u>: Reported or observed obesity in one or both parents; rapid transition across growth percentiles in infants or children; dysfunctional eating patterns: eating in response to external cues such as the time of day; eating in response to internal cues other than hunger (e.g., anxiety).

•Altered Oral Mucous Membrane

<u>Definitions</u>: The state in which an individual experiences disruptions in the tissue layers of the oral cavity.
<u>Etiology/related to factors</u>: Radiation to the head or neck; dehydration; chemical trauma (e.g., acidic foods, drugs, alcohol); mechanical trauma (e.g., ill fitting dentures, endotracheal or nasogastric tubes; NPO for more than 24 hours; ineffective oral hygiene; mouth breathing; malnutrition; infection; medications.
<u>Defining characteristics</u>: Oral pain; coated tongue; xerostomia (dry mouth); stomatitis; oral lesions or ulcers; decreased salivation; leukoplakia; oral plaque; carious teeth; halitosis.

•Altered Parenting

<u>Definition</u>: The state in which a nurturing figure(s) experiences an inability to create an environment which promotes the optimum growth and development of another human being.
<u>Etiology/related to factors</u>: Lack of available role model; physical and psychosocial abuse of nurturing figure; interruption in bonding process;mental or physical illness;limited cognitive functioning.
<u>Defining characteristics</u>: Abandonment; inattentive to infant or child needs; inappropriate caretaking behavior (toilet training, sleep, rest, feeding); history of child abuse or abandonment by primary caretaker.

•Altered Protection

<u>Definition</u>: An individual experiences a decrease in the ability to guard the self from internal or external threats such as illness or injury.
<u>Etiology/related to factors</u>: Extremes of age; inadequate nutrition; alcohol abuse; abnormal blood profiles (e.g., leukopenia, anemia); immunosuppression; drug therapies (e.g., antineoplastic, corticosteroid, anticoagulants).
<u>Defining characteristics</u>: Deficit immunity; impaired healing; altered clotting; maladaptive stress response; neurosensory alteration; chilling; perspiring; fatigue.

•Altered Role Performance

<u>Definition</u>: Disruption in the way one perceives one's role performance.
<u>Etiology/related to factors</u>: [Situational or maturational crises]; [involuntary release from employment]; [death of spouse or significant other].
<u>Defining characteristics</u>: Change in self-perception; denial of role; change in others perception of role; conflict in roles; changes in physical capacity to resume role; change in usual patterns of responsibility.

•Altered Sexuality Patterns

<u>Definition</u>: The state in which an individual expresses concern regarding his/her sexuality.
<u>Etiology/related to factors</u>: Altered body function; knowledge deficit about alternative responses to health-related transitions; lack of significant other; fear of acquiring a sexually transmitted disease.
<u>Defining characteristics</u>: Reported difficulties, limitation or changes in sexual behaviors or activities.

•Altered Thought Processes

<u>Definition</u>: [An individual experiences a disruption in cognitive operations and activities].
<u>Etiology/related to factors</u>: [Cognitive distortions]; [developmental lag]; [sensory overload]; [substance abuse].
<u>Defining characteristics</u>: Inaccurate interpretation of environment; cognitive dissonance; distractibility; memory deficit; egocentricity; hyper- or hypovigilance.

•Altered Tissue Perfusion (Specify: Renal, Cerebral, Cardiopulmonary, Gastrointestinal, or Peripheral)

<u>Definition</u>: An individual experiences a decrease in nutrition and oxygenation at the cellular level due to a deficit in capillary blood supply.
<u>Etiology/related to factors</u>: Interruption of flow, arterial; interruption of flow, venous; exchange problems; hypovolemia; hypervolemia.
<u>Defining characteristics</u>: Cold extremities; dependent blue or purple skin color; pale on elevation, color does not return on lowering of leg; diminished arterial pulsations; shining skin; lack of lanugo; slow-growing, dry brittle nails; claudication; bruits; slow healing of lesions.

•Altered Urinary Elimination

Definition: An individual experiences a disturbance in urine elimination.
Etiology/related to factors: Multiple causality, including: anatomical obstruction, sensory motor impairment, urinary tract infection.
Defining characteristics: Dysuria; frequency; hesitancy; incontinence; nocturia; retention; urgency.

•Anticipatory Grieving

Definition: [An individual or family demonstrate signs and symptoms of the grieving process in anticipation of a loss].
Etiology/related to factors: [Expectation of a loss].
Defining characteristics: Expression of distress at potential loss of significant other or object; expressions of guilt, anger, sorrow, and changes in libido; changes in eating habits; alterations in sleep patterns, activity level, communication.

•Anxiety

Definition: A vague uneasy feeling whose source is often nonspecific or unknown to the individual.
Etiology/related to factors: Unknown conflict about essential values or goals of life; threat to self-concept; threat of death; threat to or change in health status; threat to or change in role functioning; threat to or change in environment; threat to or change in interaction patterns; situational or maturational crises; interpersonal transmission or contagion.
Defining characteristics: Sympathetic stimulation such as cardiovascular excitation, superficial vasoconstriction, pupil dilation; restlessness; insomnia; poor eye contact; trembling; facial muscles taut; voice quivering; verbalizations of increased tension, fearful, feelings of inadequacy worried.

•Bathing/Hygiene Self-Care Deficit

Definition: A state in which the individual experiences an impaired ability to perform or complete bathing/hygiene activities for oneself.
Etiology/related to factors: Intolerance to activity, decreased strength and endurance; pain, discomfort; perceptual or cognitive impairment; neuromuscular impairment; musculoskeletal impairment; depression, sever anxiety.
Defining characteristics: Inability to wash body or body parts; inability to obtain or get to water source; inability to regulate temperature or flow.

•Body Image Disturbance

Definition: Disruption in the way one perceives one's body image.
Etiology/related to factors: Biophysical; cognitive or perceptual; psychosocial; cultural or spiritual.
Defining characteristics: Verbal response to actual or perceived change in structure or function such as verbalizations of fear of rejection or reaction by others; preoccupation with loss; personalization of the part by name; depersonalization of the part by impersonal pronouns; refusal to verify actual change. Nonverbal response to actual or perceived change in structure or function such as not looking at part; not touching body part; inability to estimate spatial relationship of body to environment.

•Bowel Incontinence

Definition: An individual experiences a change in normal bowel habits characterized by involuntary passage of stool.
Etiology/related to factors: [Decreased level of consciousness]; [poor sphincter control];
Defining characteristics: Involuntary passage of stool.

•Chronic Low Self-Esteem

Definition: Long standing negative self-evaluation or feelings about self or self capabilities.
Etiology/related to factors: See Self-esteem disturbance.
Defining characteristics: Long standing or chronic manifestation of the defining characteristics identified in Self-esteem disturbance.

•Chronic Pain

Definition: The individual experiences pain that continues for more than six months induration.
Etiology/related to factors: Chronic physical or psychosocial disability.
Defining characteristics: Verbal report or observed evidence of pain experienced for more than 6 months; fear of another injury; physical and social withdrawal.

•Colonic Constipation

Definition: An individual's pattern of elimination is characterized by hard, dry stool which results from a delay in passage of food residue.
Etiology/related to factors: Less than adequate fluid intake; less than adequate dietary intake; less than adequate fluid intake; immobility.
Defining characteristics: Decreased frequency; hard, dry stool; straining at stool; painful defecation; abdominal distention; palpable mass.

•Constipation

Definition: An individual experiences a change in normal bowel habits characterized by a decrease in frequency and/ or passage of hard day stools.
Etiology/related to factors: [Low roughage diet]; [low fluid intake]; [decreased activity level]; [absence of routine time for bowel movements]; [side effect of medications].
Defining characteristics: Frequency of stool less than usual pattern; hard formed stools; palpable mass; reported feeling of pressure in rectum; straining at stool; [decreased bowel sounds]; [abdominal distention].

•Decisional Conflict (Specify)

Definition: The state of uncertainty about course of action to be taken when choice among competing actions involves risk, loss, or challenge to personal life values.
Etiology/related to factors: Unclear personal values; perceived threat to value system; support system deficit.
Defining characteristics: Verbalized uncertainty about choices; vacillation between alternative choices; delayed decision making.

•Decreased Cardiac Output

Definition: A state in which the blood pumped by an individual's heart is sufficiently reduced that it is inadequate to meet the needs of the body's tissues.
Etiology/related to factors: [Side effects of medications e.g., cocaine]; [effect alcohol on the heart muscle]; [electrical alteration in rate, rhythm, conduction].
Defining characteristics: Variations in blood pressure readings; arrhythmias; fatigue; jugular vein distention; color changes, skin and mucous membranes; oliguria; decreased peripheral pulses; cold clammy skin; adventitious breath sounds (crackles); dyspnea; orthopnea.

•Defensive Coping

Definition: The state in which an individual repeatedly projects falsely positive self-evaluation based on a self-protective pattern which defends against underlying perceived threats to positive self-regard.
Etiology/related to factors: [Anxiety]; [lack of problem-solving skills]; [perceived threat to self].
Defining characteristics: Denial of obvious problems; projection of blame; rationalizes failures; grandiosity.

•Diarrhea

Definition: An individual experiences a change in normal bowel habits characterized by the frequent passage of loose, fluid, unformed stools.
Etiology/related to factors: [Food intolerance]; [medications]; [stress]; [contaminants]; [tube feedings].
Defining characteristics: Abdominal pain; cramping, increased frequency; increased frequency of bowel sounds; loose liquid stools; urgency.

•Diversional Activity Deficit

Definition: An individual experiences a decreased stimulation from or interest or engagement in recreational or leisure activities.
Etiology/related to factors: Environmental lack of diversional activity (e.g., long-term hospitalization, frequent lengthy treatments).
Defining characteristics: Client's statements regarding boredom; usual hobbies cannot be undertaken in hospital.

•Dressing/Grooming Self-Care Deficit

Definition: An impaired ability to perform or complete dressing and grooming activities for oneself.
Etiology/related to factors: Intolerance to activity, decreased strength and endurance; pain, discomfort; perceptual or cognitive impairment; neuromuscular impairment; musculoskeletal impairment; depression, severe anxiety.
Defining characteristics: Impaired ability to put on or take off necessary items of clothing; impaired ability to obtain or replace articles of clothing; impaired ability to fasten clothing; inability to maintain appearance at a satisfactory level.

•Dysfunctional Grieving

Definition: [An individual or family's grief process is extended or unresolved relating to an actual or perceived loss].
Etiology/related to factors: Actual or perceived object loss (e.g., Change in relationships; loss of a significant other, job or object).
Defining characteristics: Verbal expressions of distress at loss; denial of loss; expression of guilt; expression of unresolved issues; anger; crying; expression of feeling sad all the time; alterations in eating habits, sleep patterns, activity level; expression of alteration in libido.

•Dysreflexia

Definition: An individual with a spinal cord injury at T7 or above experiences a life threatening uninhibited sympathetic response of the nervous system to a noxious stimulus.
Etiology/related to factors: Bladder distention; bowel distention; skin irritation.
Defining characteristics: Chilling; conjunctival congestion; Horner's syndrome (contraction of the pupil, partial ptosis of the eyelid, enophthalmos and sometimes loss of sweating over the affected side of the face); paresthesia; pilomotor reflex; blurred vision; chest pain; metallic taste in mouth; nasal congestion.

•Effective Breastfeeding

Definition: The state in which a mother-infant dyad/family exhibits adequate proficiency and satisfaction with breastfeeding process.
Etiology/related to factors: Basic breastfeeding knowledge; normal breast structure; normal infant oral structure; maternal confidence.
Defining characteristics: Mother able to position infant at breast to promote a successful latch-on response; infant is content after feeding; regular and sustained suckling/swallowing at the breast; appropriate infant weight patterns for age.

•Family Coping: Potential for Growth

Definition: Effective managing of adaptive tasks by family member involved with the client's health challenge, who now is exhibiting desire and readiness for enhanced health and growth in regard to self and in relation to the client.
Etiology/related to factor: Needs sufficiently gratified and adaptive tasks effectively addressed to enable goals of self-actualization to surface.

•Fatigue

Definition: An overwhelming sustained sense of exhaustion and decreased capacity for physical and mental work.
Etiology/related to factors: Decreased or increased metabolic energy production; overwhelming psychological or emotional demands; increased energy requirements to perform activity of daily living; altered body chemistry (e.g., medications, drug withdrawal, chemotherapy).
Defining characteristics: Verbalization of an unremitting and overwhelming lack of energy; inability to maintain usual routines.

•Fear

Definition: Feeling of dread related to an identifiable source which the person validates.
Etiology/related to factors: [Lack of support system]; [lack of knowledge]; [language barrier]; [sensory impairment]; [perceived inability to control event.]
Defining characteristics: Ability to identify object of fear; [verbally expresses dread, nervousness or concern about a threatening event, person, object]; [restlessness]; [diaphoresis]; [increased heart and respiratory rate]; [increased muscle tension].

•Feeding Self-Care Deficit

Definition: An individual experiences an impaired ability to perform or complete feeding activities for oneself.
Etiology/related to factors: Intolerance to activity, decreased strength and endurance; pain, perceptual or cognitive impairment; neuromuscular impairment; musculoskeletal impairment; depression, severe anxiety.
Defining characteristics: Inability to bring food from a receptacle to the mouth.

•Fluid Volume Deficit

Definition: The state in which an individual experiences vascular, cellular, or intracellular dehydration.
Etiology/related to factors: Active fluid volume loss; failure of regulatory mechanisms.
Defining characteristics: Change in urine output; change in urine concentration; sudden weight loss or gain; decreased venous filling; hemoconcentration; change in serum sodium.

•Fluid Volume Excess

Definition: An individual experiences increased fluid retention and edema.
Etiology/related to factors: Compromised regulatory mechanism; excess fluid intake; excess sodium intake.
Defining characteristics: Edema; effusion; anasarca; weight gain; shortness of breath; orthopnea; intake greater than output; abnormal breath sounds (crackles); change in respiratory pattern; change in mental status; blood pressure changes; central venous pressure changes; jugular vein distention; changes specific gravity; azotemia; altered electrolytes; restlessness and anxiety.

•Functional Incontinence

Definition: The state in which an individual experiences an involuntary, unpredictable passage of urine.
Etiology/related to factors: Altered environment; sensory, cognitive or mobility deficits.
Defining characteristics: Urge to void or bladder contractions sufficiently strong to result in loss of urine before reaching an appropriate receptacle.

•Health Seeking Behaviors (Specify)

Definition: A state in which an individual in stable health is actively seeking ways to alter personal health habits, and/or the environment in order to move toward a higher level of health.
Etiology/related to factors: [desire to achieve an optimal state of wellness and well-being].
Defining characteristics: Expressed or observed desire to seek a higher level of wellness; unfamiliarity with wellness resources in the community; annual physical examination.

•Hopelessness

Definition: An individual sees limited or no alternatives or personal choices available and is unable to mobilize energy on own behalf.
Etiology/related to factors: Prolonged activity restriction creating isolation; failing or deteriorating physiological condition; long-term stress; abandonment; lost belief in transcendent values or God.
Defining characteristics: Passivity, decreased verbalization; decreased affect; verbal cues of despondence (e.g., "I can't").

•Hypothermia

Definition: An individual's body temperature is reduced below normal range.
Etiology/related to factors: Damage to hypothalamus; exposure to cool or cold environment; inability or decreased ability to shiver; inadequate clothing.
Defining characteristics: Reduction in body temperature below normal range; shivering; cool skin; pallor.

•Hyperthermia

Definition: An individuals's body temperature is elevated above his/her normal range.
Etiology/related to factors: Exposure to hot environment; increased metabolic rate; dehydration; medications; anesthesia; inappropriate clothing; decreased ability to perspire.
Defining characteristics: Increase in body temperature above normal range; flushed skin; warm to touch; increased respiratory rate; tachycardia; convulsions.

•Impaired Adjustment

Definition: The state in which the individual is unable to modify his/her life style or behavior in a manner consistent with a change in health status.
Etiology/related to factors: Disability requiring change in life style; inadequate support systems; impaired cognition; sensory overload.
Defining characteristics: Verbalization of nonacceptance of health status change; unsuccessful in goal-setting; [expression of anger toward others].

•Impaired Gas Exchange

Definition: The state in which the individual experiences a decreased passage of oxygen and/or carbon dioxide between the alveoli of the lungs and the vascular system.
Etiology/related to factors: Ventilation perfusion imbalance.
Defining characteristics: Confusion; somnolence; restlessness; irritability; inability to move secretions; hypercapnia; hypoxia.

•Impaired Home Maintenance Management

Definition: Inability to independently maintain a safe growth-promoting immediate environment.
Etiology/related to factors: Individual or family member disease or injury;insufficient family organization or planning; insufficient finances; unfamiliarity with community resources; impaired cognitive or emotional functioning.
Defining characteristics: Household members express difficulty in maintaining their home in a comfortable fashion; household request assistance with home maintenance; household members describe outstanding debts or financial crises. Unwashed or unavailable cooking equipment, clothes or linen; accumulation of dirt, food wastes; exhausted family members; repeated hygienic disorders, infestations, or infections.

•Impaired Physical Mobility

Definition: A state in which the individual experiences a limitation of ability for independent physical movement.
Etiology/related to factors: Intolerance to activity; decreased strength and endurance; pain or discomfort; perceptual or cognitive impairment; neuromuscular impairment; musculoskeletal impairment; depression or sever anxiety.
Defining characteristics: Inability to purposefully move within the physical environment; limited range of motion; decreased muscle strength; imposed restrictions of movement (e.g., restraints).
Functional Level Classification
0 = Completely independent
1 = Required use of equipment or device
2 = Requires help from another person, for assistance, supervision or teaching.
3 = Requires help from another person and equipment device
4 = Dependent, does not participate in activity.

•Impaired Skin Integrity

Definitions: A state in which the individual's skin is adversely altered.
Etiology/related to factors: (Environmental) hyper- or hypothermia; chemical substance; mechanical factors (shearing forces, pressure, restraint); radiation; physical immobilization. (Individual) medications; obesity or emaciation; altered metabolic state; altered circulation; altered sensation; skeletal prominence.
Defining characteristics: Disruption of skin surface; destruction of skin layers; invasion of body structures.

•Impaired Social Interaction

Definition: Insufficient or excessive quantity or ineffective quality of social exchange.
Etiology/related to factors: Communication barriers; self-concept disturbance; absence of available significant others or peers; limited physical mobility; therapeutic isolation; environmental barriers.
Defining characteristics: Verbalized or observed discomfort in social situations; verbalized or observed inability to receive or communicate a satisfying sense of belonging, caring, interest or shared history; observed use of unsuccessful social interaction behaviors; dysfunctional interactions with peers, family and or others.

•Impaired Swallowing

Definition: Decreased ability to voluntarily pass fluids and/or solids from the mouth to the stomach.
Etiology/related to factors: Neuromuscular impairment (e.g., decreased or absent gag reflex, decreased strength of muscles involved in mastication); mechanical obstruction (e.g., tracheotomy tube); fatigue; limited awareness; reddened, irritated oropharyngeal cavity.
Defining characteristics: Observed evidence of difficulty in swallowing (e.g., stasis of food in oral cavity, coughing or choking).

•Impaired Tissue Integrity

Definition: An individual experiences damage to mucous membranes, corneal, integumentary, or subcutaneous tissue.
Etiology/related to factors: Altered circulation; nutritional deficit or excess; fluid deficit or excess; irritants (chemical, thermal, mechanical).
Defining characteristics: Damaged or destroyed tissue of cornea, mucous membrane, integumentary, or subcutaneous).

•Impaired Verbal Comunication

<u>Definition</u>: An individual experiences a decreased or absent ability to use or understand language in human interaction.

<u>Etiology/related to factors</u>: Decrease in circulation to brain; physical barrier (e.g., tracheostomy); anatomical defect (e.g., cleft palate); cultural difference; [English as a second language].

<u>Defining characteristics</u>: Unable to speak dominant language; speaks or verbalizes with difficulty; does not or cannot speak; stuttering; slurring; difficulty forming words; difficulty expressing thoughts verbally; disorientation.

•Ineffective Airway Clearance

<u>Definition</u>: A state in which an individual is unable to clear secretions or obstructions from the respiratory tract to maintain airway patency.

<u>Etiology/related to factors</u>: Decreased energy/fatigue; tracheobronchial infection; obstruction; excess thick secretions; perceptual/cognitive impairment; trauma.

<u>Defining characteristics</u>: Abnormal breath sounds: crackles, wheezes; changes in rate or depth of respiration; tachypnea; cough, effective or ineffective, with or without sputum; cyanosis; dyspnea.

•Ineffective Breastfeeding

<u>Definition</u>: The state in which a mother, infant, or child experience dissatisfaction or difficulty with the breastfeeding process.

<u>Etiology/related to factors</u>: Prematurity; infant anomaly; maternal breast anomaly; maternal anxiety or ambivalence.

<u>Defining characteristics</u>: Unsatisfactory breastfeeding process; actual or perceived inadequate milk supply; infant inability to attach on to maternal breast correctly; insufficient emptying of each breast per feeding; persistence of sore nipples beyond the first week of breastfeeding.

•Ineffective Breathing Pattern

<u>Definition</u>: The state in which an individual's inhalation and or exhalation pattern does not enable adequate pulmonary inflation or emptying.

<u>Etiology/related to factors</u>: Neuromuscular impairment; pain, musculoskeletal impairment; perception or cognitive impairment; anxiety; decreased energy or fatigue.

<u>Defining characteristics</u>: Dyspnea; shortness of breath; tachypnea; fremitus; abnormal arterial blood gases; cyanosis; cough; nasal flaring; respiratory depth changes; purse-lip breathing; prolonged expiratory phase, increased anteroposterior diameter; use of accessory muscles; altered chest excursion.

•Ineffective Denial

<u>Definition</u>: A conscious or unconscious attempt to disavow the knowledge or meaning of an event to reduce anxiety or fear to the detriment of health.

<u>Etiology/related to factors</u>: [Fear]; [substance abuse]; [perceived threat to self].

<u>Defining characteristics</u>: Delays seeking health care to the detriment of health; does not perceive personal relevance of symptoms or danger; uses home remedies to relieve symptoms.

•Ineffective Family Coping: Compromised

<u>Definition</u>: A usually supportive primary person is providing insufficient, ineffective, or compromised support, comfort, assistance, or encouragement which may be needed by the client to manage or master adaptive tasks related to his or her health challenge.

<u>Etiology/related to factors</u>: Progression of disease exhausts the supportive capacity of significant other; temporary family disorganization and role changes; incorrect information or understanding by a primary person.

<u>Defining characteristics</u>: Client expresses a concern about significant other's response to his or her health problem; significant other confirms inadequate understanding of knowledge base which interferes with effective supportive behaviors; significant other withdraws into limited communication with client at the time of need.

•Ineffective Family Coping: Disabling

<u>Definition</u>: Behavior of significant person that disables his or her own capacities and the client's capacities to effectively address tasks essential to either person's adaptation to the health challenge.

<u>Etiology/related to factors</u>: Significant person with chronically unexpressed feelings of guilt, anxiety, hostility, despair; arbitrary handling of family's resistance to treatment.

<u>Defining characteristics</u>: Neglectful care of client in regard to basic human needs or illness treatment; distortion of reality regarding the client's health problem; abandonment; hostility.

•Ineffective Individual Coping

Definition: Impairment of adaptive behaviors and problem-solving abilities of a person in meeting life's demands and roles.
Etiology/related to factors: Situational crises; maturational crises; personal vulnerability.
Defining characteristics: Verbalization of inability to cope or inability to ask for help; inability to meet basic needs; inability to problem-solve; high rate of accidents.

•Ineffective Thermoregulation

Definition: The individual's temperature fluctuated between hypothermia and hyperthermia.
Etiology/related to factors: Trauma or illness; immaturity; aging; fluctuating environmental temperature.
Defining characteristics: Fluctuation in body temperature above or below the normal range. See hypothermia and hyperthermia.

•Knowledge Deficit

Definition: [An individual is unable to verbalize information and demonstrate skills necessary to achieve a state of wellness and well-being].
Etiology/related to factors: Lack of exposure; lack of recall; information misinterpretation; cognitive limitation; lack of interest in learning; unfamiliarity with information resources.
Defining characteristics: Verbalization of the problem; inaccurate follow-through of instruction; inaccurate performance of test; inappropriate or exaggerated behavior (e.g., hostile).

•Non-Compliance (Specify)

Definition: A person's informed decision not to adhere to a therapeutic recommendation.
Etiology/related to factors: Patient value system: health beliefs, cultural influences, spiritual values; client-provider relationships.
Defining characteristics: Behavior indicative of failure to adhere; failure to keep appointments; [failure to follow therapeutic regime].

•Pain

Definition: An individual experiences and reports the presence of severe discomfort or an uncomfortable sensation.
Etiology/related to factors: Injury agents (e.g., biological, chemical, physical, psychological).
Defining characteristics: Communication verbally of pain descriptors; guarding behavior; self-focusing; narrowed focus; distraction behavior (e.g., moaning, crying, pacing, seeking out other people, restlessness); facial mask of pain (e.g., eyes lack luster, fixed or scattered movement, grimace); alteration in muscle tone; autonomic responses not seen in chronic stable pain (e.g., diaphoresis, blood pressure and pulse change, pupillary dilation, increased or decreased respiratory rate).

•Parental Role Conflict

Definition: The state in which a parent experiences role confusion and conflict in response to crisis.
Etiology/related to factors: Separation from child due to chronic illness; change in marital status.
Defining characteristics: Parent expresses concern of inadequacy to provide for child's physical and emotional needs; demonstrated disruption in care taking routines.

•Perceived Constipation

Definition: An individual makes a self-diagnosis of constipation and ensures a daily bowel movement through abuse of laxatives, enemas, and suppositories.
Etiology/related to factors: Cultural and family health beliefs; faculty appraisal; impaired thought processes.
Defining characteristics: Expectation of a daily movement with the resulting overuse of laxatives, enemas, and suppositories; expected passage of stool at same time every day.

•Personal Identity Disturbance

Definition: Inability to distinguish between self and oneself.
Etiology/related to factors: [Disintegration of ego boundaries]; [disintegration of thought processes]; [unmet dependency needs]; [retarded ego development].
Defining characteristics: [Extreme mood changes]; [inability to define self-boundaries]; [inability to give direction to life or set goals]; [presence of more than one personality within the individual].

•Post-Trauma Response

Definition: An individual experiencing a sustained painful response to an overwhelming traumatic event(s).
Etiology/related to factors: Disasters, wars, epidemics, rape, assault, torture, catastrophic illness or accident.
Defining characteristics: Reexperience of the traumatic event which may be identified in cognitive, affective, and/or sensory motor activities (e.g., flashbacks, repetitive nightmares, excessive verbalization of the traumatic event, verbalization of survival guilt).

•Potential Activity Intolerance

Definition: Individual is at risk of experiencing insufficient physiological or psychological energy to endure or complete required or desired daily activities.
Related to the presence of risk factors: History of previous intolerance; deconditioned status; presence of circulatory or respiratory problems; inexperience with the activity; [sedentary lifestyle].

•Potential Altered Body Temperature

Definition: The individual is at risk for failure to maintain body temperature within normal range.
Related to the presence of risk factors: Extremes of age; extremes of weight; exposure to extremes in environmental temperature; dehydration; illness or trauma affecting temperature regulation.

•Potential Altered Parenting

Definition: [The presence of risk factors that may interfere with the nurturing figure's ability to promote optimum growth and development of another human being].
Related to the presence of risk factors: Lack of available role model; lack of support from significant other; unmet emotional needs of parenting figures.

•Potential for Aspiration

Definition: An individual is at risk for entry of gastrointestinal secretions, oropharyngeal secretions, or solids or fluids into tracheobronchial passages.
Related to the presence of risk factors: Reduced level of consciousness; depressed cough and gag reflexes; presence of tracheostomy or endotracheal tube; tube feedings; impaired swallowing; wired jaws.

•Potential for Disuse Syndrome

Definition: An individual is at risk for deterioration of body systems as the result of prescribed or unavoidable musculoskeletal inactivity.
Related to the presence of risk factors: Paralysis; mechanical immobilization; severe pain; altered level of consciousness.

•Potential Fluid Volume Deficit

Definition: The state in which an individual is at risk for experiencing vascular, cellular, or intracellular dehydration.
Related to the presence of risk factors: Lack of access to fluids; medications (e.g., diuretics); immobility; hypermetabolic state; excessive losses through normal routes (e.g., diarrhea); excessive losses through abnormal routes (e.g., indwelling tubes); failure to drink sufficient amounts fluid.

•Potential Impaired Skin Integrity

Definition: A state in which the individual's skin is at risk of being adversely altered.
Related to the presence of risk factors: (Environmental) hypo- or hyperthermia; chemical substances; mechanical factors; radiation; physical immobilization; excretions or secretions. (Individual) altered metabolic state; obesity or emaciation; altered sensation; skeletal prominence; psychogenic; immunologic.

•Potential for Infection

Definition: An individual is at increased risk for invasion by pathogenic organisms.
Related to the presence of risk factors: Inadequate primary defenses (e.g., broken skin); inadequate secondary defense (e.g., decreased hemoglobin, immunosuppression, chronic disease); invasive procedures; malnutrition; trauma; lack of knowledge to avoid exposure to pathogens.

•Potential for Injury

Definition: An individual is at risk of injury as a result of environmental conditions interacting with the individual's adaptive and defensive resources.
Related to the presence of risk factors: Internal (broken skin, immobility, disoriented, overdose CNS depressants, pharmacologic effects of anesthesia); external (immunization level of the community; environmental pollutants).

•Potential for Poisoning

Definition: Accentuated risk of accidental exposure to or ingestion of drugs or dangerous products in doses sufficient to cause poisoning.
Related to the presence of risk factors: (Individual) reduced vision; verbalization of occupational setting without adequate safeguards; lack of drug education; cognitive or emotional difficulties. (Environmental) large supplies of drugs in house; chemical contamination of food and water; presence of atmospheric pollutants.

•Potential for Suffocation

Definition: Accentuated risk of accidental suffocation (inadequate air available for inhalation).
Related to the presence of risk factors: Reduced olfactory sensation; reduced motor abilities; lack of safety education and precautions (smoking in bed); cognitive or emotional difficulties; eating large mouthfuls of food.

•Potential for Trauma

Definition: Accentuated risk of accidental tissue injury (e.g., wound, burn, fracture).
Related to the presence of risk factors: (Individual) weakness; poor vision; balancing difficulties; reduced tactile sensation; reduced large or small muscle coordination; reduced hand-eye coordination; lack of safely education; cognitive or emotional difficulties. (Environmental) slippery floors; contact with intense cold; overexposure to radiotherapy.

•Potential For Violence: Self-Directed or Directed at Others

Definition: An individual experiences behaviors that can be physically harmful either to the self or others.
Etiology/related to factors: Antisocial character; battered women; catatonic excitement; child abuse; manic excitement; organic brain syndrome; panic state; rage reactions; suicidal behavior; toxic reactions to mediation.
Defining characteristics: Body language (e.g., clenched fists, facial muscles taut, rigid posture); hostile threatening verbalizations (e.g., boasting of abuse to others); increased motor activity (e.g., pacing); overt and aggressive acts (e.g., goal-directed destruction of objects in environment); possession of destructive means (e.g., gun, knife).

•Powerlessness

Definition: Perception that ones's own action will not significantly affect an outcome; a perceived lack of control over a current situation or immediate happening.
Etiology/related to factors: Health care environment; interpersonal interaction; illness-related regimen; life-style of helplessness.
Defining characteristics: Verbal expressions of having no control or influence over situation; verbal expressions of having no control or influence over outcome; verbal expressions of having no control over self-care; depression over physical deterioration which occurs despite client compliance with regimens; apathy.

•Rape-Trauma Syndrome

Definition: Forced violent sexual penetration against the victim's will and consent. The trauma syndrome that develops from this attack or attempted attack includes an acute phase of disorganization of the victim's life-style and a long-term process of reorganization of life-style.
Etiology/related to factors: [Sexual abuse].
Defining characteristics: Acute phase includes emotional reactions such as anger, embarrassment, fear of physical violence and death, humiliation, revenge, self-blame; multiple physical symptoms such as gastrointestinal irritability, genitourinary discomfort, muscle tension, sleep pattern disturbance. Long-term reactions include changes in life-style such as change in residence, repetitive nightmares and phobias, seeking family support, seeking social network support.

•Rape-Trauma Syndrome: Compound Reaction

<u>Definition</u>: See Rape-trauma syndrome.
<u>Etiology/related to</u>: [Sexual abuse].
<u>Defining characteristics</u>: See Rape-trauma syndrome. Reactivated symptoms of such previous conditions such as physical illness, psychiatric illness, reliance on alcohol or drugs.

•Rape-Trauma Syndrome: Silent Reaction

<u>Definition</u>: See Rape-trauma syndrome.
<u>Etiology/related to factors</u>: [Sexual abuse]
<u>Defining characteristics</u>: Abrupt changes in relationships with men; increase in nightmares; increased anxiety during interview (e.g., blocking of associations, long periods of silence, minor stuttering); pronounced changes in sexual behavior; no verbalization of the occurrence of rape; sudden onset of phobic reactions.

•Reflex Incontinence

<u>Definition</u>: The state in which an individual experiences an involuntary loss of urine, occurring at somewhat predictable intervals when a specific bladder volume is reached.
<u>Etiology/related to factors</u>: Neurological impairment (e.g., spinal cord lesion which interferes with conduction of cerebral messages above the level of the reflex arc).
<u>Defining characteristics</u>: No awareness of bladder filling; no urge to void or feelings of bladder fullness; uninhabited bladder contraction or spasm at regular intervals.

•Self-Esteem Disturbance

<u>Definition</u>: Negative self-evaluation or feelings about self or self-capabilities, which may be directly or indirectly expressed.
<u>Etiology/related to factors</u>: [History of physical sexual or verbal abuse]: [disintegrated thought processes]; [unmet dependency needs]; [retarded ego development]; [dysfunctional family support system].
<u>Defining characteristics</u>: Self-negating verbalization; expressions of shame or guilt; evaluates self as unable to deal with events; rationalizes away or rejects positive feedback and exaggerates negative feedback about self.

•Sensory/Perceptual Alterations (Specify: Visual, Auditory, Kinesthetic, Gustatory, Tactile, Olfactory)

<u>Definition</u>: An individual experiences a change in the amount or patterning of oncoming stimuli accompanied by a diminished, exaggerated, distorted or impaired response to such stimuli.
<u>Etiology/related to factors</u>: Altered environmental stimuli; altered sensory reception, transmission or integration; chemical alteration from electrolyte imbalance or medications; psychological stress.
<u>Defining characteristics</u>: Disoriented to time, place or person; altered abstraction; altered conceptualization; change in problem-solving abilities; reported or measured change in sensory acuity; change in behavior pattern; altered communication patterns.

•Sexual Dysfunction

<u>Definition</u>: A change in sexual function that is viewed as unsatisfying, unrewarding, inadequate.
<u>Etiology/related to factors</u>: Biopsychosocial alteration of sexuality; physical abuse; lack of significant other; altered body structure; disease process.
<u>Defining characteristics</u>: Verbalization of problem; actual or perceived limitation imposed by disease; change of interest in self and others.

•Situational Low Self-Esteem

<u>Definition</u>: Negative self-evaluation or feelings about self which develop in response to a loss or change in an individual who previously had a positive self-evaluation.
<u>Etiology/related to factors</u>: [Loss of employment]; [change in family support system]; [change in cognitive processes]; [change in physical abilities].
<u>Defining characteristics</u>: Episodic occurrence of negative self-appraisal in response to life events in a person with a previous positive self-evaluation; verbalization of negative feelings about the self such as hopelessness, uselessness; [perceived inability to make further contributions to family and community].

•Sleep Pattern Disturbance

<u>Definition</u>: Disruption of sleep time causes discomfort or interferes with desired life-style.
<u>Etiology/related to factors</u>: Sensory alterations due to illness, psychological stress; environmental changes.
<u>Defining characteristics</u>: Verbal complaints of difficulty falling asleep; awakening earlier or later than desired; interrupted sleep; verbal complaints of not feeling well-rested; lethargy; ptosis of eyelid; dark circles under eyes; frequent yawning; changes in posture; thick speech with mispronunciation and incorrect words.

•Social Isolation

<u>Definition</u>: Aloneness experienced by the individual and perceived as imposed by others and as a negative or threatened state.
<u>Etiology/related to factors</u>: Delay in accomplishing developmental tasks; immature interests; alterations in physical appearance; alterations in mental status; unaccepted social behavior.
<u>Defining characteristics</u>: Absence of supportive significant others; sad dull affect; uncommunicative; no eye contact; expresses feelings of aloneness imposed by others; expresses feelings of rejection.

•Spiritual Distress (Distress of the Human Spirit)

<u>Definition</u>: Disruption in the life principle which pervades a person's entire being and which integrates and transcends one's biological and psychosocial nature.
<u>Etiology/related to factors</u>: Separation from religious or cultural ties; challenged belief and value system.
<u>Defining characteristics</u>: Expresses concern with meaning of life, death and belief systems; anger toward God; questions meaning of suffering.

•Stress Incontinence

<u>Definition</u>: The state in which an individual experiences a loss of urine of less than 50 ml occurring with increased abdominal pressure.
<u>Etiology/related to factors</u>: Degenerative changes in pelvic muscles and structural supports associated with increased age: high intra-abdominal pressures (e.g., obesity); incompetent bladder outlet; overdistention between voiding; weak pelvic muscles and structural supports.
<u>Defining characteristics</u>: Reported or observed dribbling with increased abdominal pressure; urinary urgency; urinary frequency (more often that every 2 hours).

•Toileting Self-Care Deficit

<u>Definition</u>: An impaired ability to perform or complete toileting activities for oneself.
<u>Etiology/related to factors</u>: Impaired transfer ability; impaired mobility status; intolerance to activity, decreased strength and endurance; pain, discomfort; perceptual or cognitive impairment; neuromuscular impairment; musculoskeletal impairment; depression, severe anxiety.
<u>Defining characteristics</u>: Unable to get to toilet or commode; unable to sit on or rise from toilet or commode; unable to manipulate clothing for toileting; unable to carry out proper toilet hygiene; unable to flush toilet or commode.

•Total Incontinence

<u>Definition</u>: The state in which an individual experiences a continuous and unpredictable loss of urine.
<u>Etiology/related to factors</u>: Neuropathy preventing transmission of reflex indicating bladder fullness; neurological dysfunction causing triggering of micturition at unpredictable times; independent contraction of detrusor reflex due to surgery; trauma or disease affecting spinal cord nerves; anatomic (fistula).
<u>Defining characteristics</u>: Constant flow of urine occurs at unpredictable times without distention or uninhibited bladder contraction or spasms; unsuccessful incontinence refractory treatments; nocturia.

•Unilateral Neglect

<u>Definition</u>: An individual is perceptually unaware of or inattentive to one side of the body.
<u>Etiology/related to factors</u>: Effects of disturbed perceptual abilities (e.g., hemianopsia, one-sided blindness; neurologic illness or trauma).
<u>Defining characteristics</u>: Consistent inattention to stimuli on an affected side.

•Urge Incontinence

<u>Definition</u>: The state in which an individual experiences involuntary passage of urine occurring soon after a strong sense of urgency to void.

<u>Etiology/related to factors</u>: Decreased bladder capacity; irritation of bladder stretch receptors causing spasm e.g., bladder infection); alcohol; caffeine; increased fluids; increased urine concentration; overdistention of bladder.

<u>Defining characteristics</u>: Urinary urgency; frequency (voiding more often than every 2 hours); bladder contracture or spasms.

•Urinary Retention

<u>Definition</u>: The individual experiences incomplete emptying of the bladder.

<u>Etiology/related to factors</u>: High urethral pressure caused by weak detrusor; inhibition of reflex arc; strong sphincter; blockage.

<u>Defining characteristics</u>: Bladder distention; small, frequent voiding or absence of urine output.

Source: North American Diagnosis Association. (1990). <u>Taxonomy I-REVISED 1990.</u> St. Louis: North American Nursing Diagnosis

Appendix E: Nursing Diagnoses Grouped by Functional Health Patterns

•Pattern I: Health Perception-Health Management

Altered Health Maintenance
Altered Protection
Health-Seeking Behaviors (specify)
Noncompliance (specify)
Potential for Infection
Potential for Injury
Potential for Poisoning
Potential for Suffocation
Potential for Trauma

•Pattern 2: Nutritional-Metabolic

Altered Nutrition: Less Than Body Requirements
Altered Nutrition: More Than Body Requirements
Altered Nutrition: Potential for More Than Body
  Requirements.
Altered Oral Mucous Membranes
Effective Breastfeeding
Fluid Volume Deficit
Fluid Volume Excess
Hyperthermia
Hypothermia
Impaired Skin Integrity
Impaired Swallowing
Impaired Tissue Integrity
Ineffective Breastfeeding
Ineffective Thermoregulation
Potential for Altered Body Temperature
Potential for Aspiration
Potential Fluid Volume Deficit
Potential for Impaired Skin Integrity

•Pattern 3: Elimination

Altered Urinary Elimination Pattern
Bowel Incontinence
Colonic Constipation
Constipation
Diarrhea
Functional Incontinence
Perceived Constipation
Reflex Incontinence
Stress Incontinence
Total Incontinence
Urge Incontinence
Urinary Retention

•Pattern 4: Activity-Exercise

Activity Intolerance
Altered Growth and Development
Altered Tissue Perfusion (Specify: Renal, Cerebral,
  Cardiopulmonary, Gastrointestinal, Peripheral)
Bathing/Hygiene Self-Care Deficit
Decreased Cardiac Output
Diversional Activity Deficit
Dressing/Grooming Self-Care Deficit
Dysreflexia
Fatigue
Feeding Self-Care Deficit
Impaired Home Maintenance Management
Impaired Physical Mobility
Ineffective Airway Clearance
Ineffective Breathing Pattern
Impaired Gas Exchange
Potential Activity Intolerance
Potential for Disuse Syndrome
Toileting Self-Care Deficit

•Pattern 5: Sleep-Rest

Sleep Pattern Disturbance

•Pattern 6: Cognitive-Perceptual

Altered Thought Processes
Chronic Pain
Decisional Conflict (specify)
Knowledge Deficit (specify)
Pain
Sensory/Perceptual Alterations (specify: Visual,
  Auditory, Kinesthetic, Gustatory, Tactile, Olfactory)
Unilateral Neglect

•Pattern 7: Self-Perception/Self-Concept

Anxiety
Body image Disturbance
Chronic low Self-Esteem
Fear
Hopelessness
Personal Identity Disturbance
Powerlessness
Self-esteem Disturbance
Situational Low Self-Esteem

•**Pattern 8: Role-Relationship**

Altered Family Processes
Altered Parenting
Altered Role Performance
Anticipatory Grieving
Dysfunctional Grieving
Impaired Social Interaction
Impaired Verbal Communication
Parental Role Conflict
Potential for Altered Parenting
Potential for Violence: Self-Directed or Directed
  at Others
Social Isolation

•**Pattern 9: Sexuality-Reproductive**

Altered Sexuality Patterns
Rape-Trauma Syndrome
Rape-Trauma Syndrome: Compound Reaction
Rape-Trauma Syndrome: Silent Reaction
Sexual Dysfunction

•**Pattern 10: Coping-Stress-Tolerance**

Defensive Coping
Family Coping: Potential for Growth
Impaired Adjustment
Ineffective Denial
Ineffective Family Coping: Disabling
Ineffective Family Coping: Compromised
Ineffective Individual Coping
Post-Trauma Response

•**Pattern 11: Value-Belief**

Spiritual Distress (Distress of the Human Spirit)

Used with permission from: Gordon, M. (1989). Manual of Nursing Diagnosis, New York: McGraw-Hill.

Appendix F: Nursing Diagnoses Grouped by Diagnostic Divisions

•Diagnostic Division #1: Activity/Rest

Activity Intolerance
Diversional Activity Deficit
Dysreflexia
Fatigue
Potential Activity Intolerance
Sleep Pattern Disturbance

•Diagnostic Division #2: Circulation

Altered Tissue Perfusion (Specify: Renal, Cerebral, Cardiopulmonary, Gastrointestinal, Peripheral)
Decreased Cardiac Output

•Diagnostic Division #3: Elimination

Altered Urinary Elimination
Bowel Incontinence
Colonic Constipation
Constipation
Diarrhea
Functional Incontinence
Perceived Constipation
Reflex Incontinence
Stress Incontinence
Total Incontinence
Urge Incontinence
Urinary Retention

•Diagnostic Division #4: Emotional Reactions

Anticipatory Grieving
Anxiety
Body Image Disturbance
Chronic Low Self-Esteem
Decisional Conflict (Specify)
Defensive Coping
Dysfunctional Grieving
Fear
Hopelessness
Impaired Adjustment
Ineffective Denial
Ineffective Individual Coping
Personal Identity Disturbance
Post-Trauma Response
Powerlessness
Rape-Trauma Syndrome
Rape-Trauma Syndrome: Compound Reaction
Rape-Trauma Syndrome: Silent Reaction
Self-Esteem Disturbance
Situational Low Self-Esteem
Spiritual Distress (Distress of the Human Spirit)

•Diagnostic Division #5: Food/Fluid

Altered Nutrition: Less Than Body Requirements
Altered Nutrition: More Than Body Requirements
Altered Nutrition: Potential for More Than Body Requirements
Altered Oral Mucous Membrane
Effective Breastfeeding
Feeding Self-Care Deficit
Fluid Volume Deficit
Fluid Volume Excess
Impaired Swallowing
Ineffective Breastfeeding
Potential Fluid Volume Deficit

•Diagnostic Division #6: Hygiene

Bathing/Hygiene Self-Care Deficit
Dressing/Grooming Self-Care Deficit
Toileting Self-Care Deficit

•Diagnostic Division #7: Neurologic

Altered Thought Processes
Impaired Verbal Communication
Sensory/Perceptual Alterations (Specify: Visual, Auditory, Kinesthetic, Gustatory, Tactile, Olfactory)
Unilateral Neglect

•Diagnostic Division #8: Pain

Chronic Pain
Pain

•Diagnostic Division #9: Relationship Alterations

Altered Family Processes
Altered Parenting
Altered Role Performance
Family Coping: Potential for Growth
Impaired Social Interaction
Ineffective Family Coping: Disabling
Ineffective Family Coping: Compromised
Parental Role Conflict
Potential Altered Parenting
Social Isolation

•Diagnostic Division #10: Safety

Altered Health Maintenance
Altered Protection
Health Seeking Behaviors (Specify)
Hyperthermia
Hypothermia
Impaired Home Maintenance Management
Impaired Physical Mobility
Impaired Skin Integrity
Impaired Tissue Integrity
Ineffective Thermoregulation
Potential for Altered Body Temperature
Potential for Aspiration
Potential for Disuse Syndrome
Potential Impaired Skin Integrity
Potential for Infection
Potential for Injury
Potential for Poisoning
Potential for Suffocation
Potential for Trauma
Potential for Violence: Self-Directed or Directed
  at Others

•Diagnostic Division #11: Sexuality

Altered Sexuality Patterns
Sexual Dysfunction

•Diagnostic Division #12: Teaching/Learning

Altered Growth and Development
Knowledge Deficit (Specify)
Noncompliance (Specify)

•Diagnostic Division #13: Ventilation

Impaired Gas Exchange
Ineffective Airway Clearance
Ineffective Breathing Pattern

Used with permission. Modified from: Doenges, M., and Moorhouse, M., (1989). Nurses Pocket Guide: Nursing Diagnoses with Interventions, 2nd Edition. Philadelphia: Davis.

Appendix G: List of Measurable Verbs and Criteria

Measurable verbs reflect the client's and nurse's actions that are seen, heard, felt or smelled. The list is a guide and not conclusive. Meaurable verbs are written in the outcome criteria, nursing orders, and nurses notes.

See	Hear	Feel
ambulate	auscultate	feel
assess	communicate	finger
cough	consult	handle
deep breath	delegate	palpate
demonstrate	describe	stroke
document	discuss	touch
drink	explain	
eat	identify	
examine	list	Smell
exercise	listen	emit
expectorate	participate	inhale
implement	percuss	smell
measure	refer	sniff
monitor	respond	whiff
observe	reinforce	
perform	reiterate	
record	report	
redemonstrate	review	
turn	state	
wash	teach	

Nonspecific Verbs: Nonspecific verbs are not measurable. Avoid using in the outcome criteria, nursing orders and nurses notes.

allow	fair	let
alter	frequent	limit
do	get	permit
employ	good	poor
enable	have	put
encourage	know	restrict
ensure	inadequate	try
facilitate	learn	use

Examples of criteria: Criteria serve as gauges of the client's progress in achieving the outcomes. The list is not conclusive.

accurately	safely	with assistance
down the hall and back	unassisted	without falling
independently	while awake	within normal limits
realistically	willingly	5 min every hour

Appendix H: List of Normal Values: Blood, Urine, Stool

This list of normal values contains information to answer the exercises in case study #1 and case study #2. The list is not conclusive. Refer to other resources for additional information.

Laboratory Value Abbreviations

< = less than	mEq = milliequivalent	mL=milliliter
> = more than	dL = deciliter	mg = milligram
g = gram	U = unit	uL = microliter
L = liter		

Chemistries

Source of specimen: serum, plasma, whole blood

Laboratory Tests	**Normal Value**
Albumin	3.5-5.0 g/dL
Blood urea nitrogen	See urea nitrogen
Calcium (Ca++)	9-11 mg/dL
Carbon dioxide (CO2 content)	20-30 mEq/L
Chloride (Cl-)	95-105 mEq/L
Cholesterol	150-270 mg/dL varies with age
Creatinine	0.5-1.5 mg/dL
Glucose, fasting	70-120 mg/dL
Potassium (K+)	3.5-5.5 mEq/L
Sodium (Na+)	135-145 mEq/L
Transaminase: Serum glutamic-oxaloacetic (SGOT)	15-45 U/L
Urea nitrogen (BUN)	10-30 mg/dL

Hematology

Red blood cells (RBC)	Male: 4.5-6.0 million/uL (mm3)
	Female: 4.0-5.0 million/uL (mm3)
Erythrocyte sedimentation rate (ERS)	Male: <15mm/h
	Female: <20 mm/h
Hematocrit (Hct)	Male: 40-54%
	Female: 38-47%
Hemoglobin (Hbg)	Male: 13.5-18.0 g/dL
	Female: 12.0-16.0 g/dL
Prothrombin time (PT)	12-15 seconds (s) Values depend on reagent used
White blood cell (WBC)	5000-10,000/uL (mm3) count

Serology-Immunology

Human immunosuppressive virus (HIV)	Negative
Rheumatoid arthritis factor (RA factor)	Negative or titer <1:20
VDRL	Nonreactive

Toxicology of Common Drugs

Salicylate level	Negative. Therapeutic level: 15-30 mg/dL

Characteristics of Normal Feces

Color	Brown
Consistency	Formed; moist
Odor	Aromatic; affected by ingested food
Frequency	Varies form 1-3 movements per day to once every 3 days
Shape	Cylindrical
Amount	100-400 g per day (varies with diet)
Fat content	<6 g/24h
Mucus	Negative
Blood	Negative
Pus	Negative
Parasites	Negative

Characteristics of Normal Urine

Amount in 24 hours	1200-1500 ml
Color	Straw, amber
Consistency	Clear liquid
Odor	Faint aromatic
Sterility	No microorganisms present
pH	4.5-8
Specific gravity	1.003-1.030
Glucose	Negative
Ketone bodies (acetone)	Negative
Blood	Negative

Diagnostic Studies

X-Ray Findings	
Chest	Negative
Bones	Joint spaces within normal limits. Negative for bony erosion, cartilage loss and cysts
Electrocardiogram (ECG)	Normal sinus rhythm
Mammogram	Negative for masses
Skin test	Negative for allergens

Appendix I: Physical Assessment

The following physical assessment findings are intended for use in the workbook exercises. The list is not conclusive. Refer to additional resources if necessary.

General Survey: Appears stated age. Sex. Race. Responds appropriately. Clean; neatly groomed. Moves without difficulty. No signs of distress such as facial grimacing, labored breathing, continual shifting of feet.

Skin: Normal skin color depends on the client's race. Uniformity of color over body. Moist. Skin temperature warm; relatively uniform over the body. Skin turgor: skin returns immediately to normal shape after being lifted, pinched and released. Skin smooth, soft; moves freely over underlying structures. No lesions. No edema. No odor. Intact.

Hair: Evenly distributed; texture varies from fine to coarse. No infestations. No flaking scalp.

Nails: Smooth texture; no clubbing or ridges. Nail bed color varies from pink to black pigmentation depending on race. No cyanosis or pallor. Blanch test: nail bed capillaries blanched when pressed and color quickly returns when pressure released. Intact tissue surrounding nail beds. Nails well groomed.

Head, Eyes, Ear, Nose and Throat: Head: Symmetrical; scalp smooth; no lesions; facial features symmetrical at rest and with movement. Temporomandibular joint (TMJ) fully movable without pain or crepitation; TMJ opening 3 to 6 cm.

Eyes: Pupils equal, round, reactive to light and accommodation (PERRLA); Extraocular movements (EOMs) intact. Conjunctiva clear; sclera white.

Ears: Hears whispered word at two feet (60 cm) bilaterally. Auricles intact bilaterally; canals clear; tympanic membranes intact and without scarring.

Nose: Symmetrical, patent, bilaterally; mucous membranes moist, intact with no discharge. Identifies odors accurately.

Mouth/throat: Mucous membrane pink/brown pigmentation in blacks, moist and intact; 32 adult teeth. Uvula midline; active gag reflex. No lesions, areas of irritation or erosion noted in oral cavity.

Neck: Trachea midline; no palpable nodes. Thyroid not palpable; full range of motion. Carotid pulse is strong, regular bilaterally and without bruits. No jugular venous distention. Equal strength sternocleidomastoid and trapezius muscles; not taut.

Pulmonary: Anteroposterior (AP) diameter of thorax 1:2. Expansion full and equal bilaterally. Lungs clear to percussion and auscultation. Respirations regular rhythm.

Breast: Rounded shape; small, medium or large nipple. Symmetrical. Skin, smooth, intact. Nipple everted, no discharge or lesions. No swelling in axillae. No tenderness, masses or nodules.

Cardiovascular: Point of maximal impulse (PMI) palpable at 5th intercostal space in midclavicular line. Apical pulse regular rhythm. No extra heart sound; no murmurs noted.

Peripheral/Vascular: No edema lower extremities.
Extremities warm to touch. Blanch test: nail bed capillaries blanched when pressed and color quickly returned when pressure released.

Peripheral Pulse Scale

0-Absent	3-Slightly diminished
1-Markedly diminished	4-Normal
2-Moderately diminished	

Abdomen: Symmetrical. Positive bowel sounds all quadrants. No masses, no tenderness on palpation. No bruits. Soft, nondistended.

Musculoskeletal: Equal strength bilaterally. Firm hand grasp. Full range of motion of hands, wrists, elbows, shoulders, spine, hips, knees and ankles. No crepitation or swelling. Even gait; balanced. No joint pain or tenderness. No abnormal curvature spine.

Grading Muscle Strength

Scale	% Normal Strength	Characteristics
0	0	Complete paralysis
1	10	No movement. Contraction of muscle is palpable or visible.
2	25	Full muscle movement against gravity, with support.
3	50	Normal movement against gravity.
4	75	Normal full movement against gravity and against minimal resistance.
5	100	Normal strength. Normal full movement against gravity and against full resistance.

Normal Range of Joint Motion

Joint Movement	Normal Range Degrees
Shoulders	
Abduction: Moves arm laterally from side position to above head, palm facing outermost	180
Elbow	
Flexion: Brings lower arm forward and upward toward shoulder	150
Wrist	
Flexion: Brings fingers of hand toward inner part of forearm	80-90
Extension: Straightens wrist from flexed position	80-90
Hyperextension: Bends fingers back as far as wrist permits	70-90
Abduction: Bends wrist to thumb side while palm faces upward	0-20
Adduction: Bends wrist toward fifth finger side, palm facing upward	30-50

> **Normal Range of Joint Motion (continued from previous page)**
> **Hand and Finger**
> <u>Flexion</u>: Makes a fist　　　　　　　　　　　　　　90
> <u>Extension</u>: Straightens fingers　　　　　　　　　90
> <u>Hyperextension</u>: Bends fingers hand　　　　　　30
> back as far as possible
> <u>Abduction</u>: Spreads fingers apart　　　　　　　20
> <u>Adduction</u>: Brings fingers together from　　　20
> abducted position

<u>Neurological</u>:　　Mental status: Alert, oriented to time, place, person. Remote and recent memory intact. Coordinated movements, upright posture, steady gait, and balance.
Cranial Nerves: Nerves I-XII intact.
Sensory: Feels and identifies correct location of soft touch bilaterally. Ability identify tastes accurately.

<u>Anus/Rectal</u>:　　Ability contract anal sphincter. Rectal exam negative for masses or lesions.

<u>Genitalia</u>:　　Penis nontender; no discharge or lesions. Testes nontender; no pitting. Negative for inguinal and femoral hernias. No vaginal discharge.

Appendix J: Vital Signs, Height, and Weight

Average Vital Signs by Age

Age	Temp.	Pulse Per Min	Respirations Per Min	BP
18 and over	37.0C (98.6F)	70-75	15-20	120/80
65 and over	36.0C (96.8F)	70-75	15-20	140/90

Height-Weight Tables,* Metropolitan 1983

Men					Women				
Height		Small	Medium	Large	Height		Small	Medium	Large
Feet	Inches	Frame	Frame	Frame	Feet	Inches	Frame	Frame	Frame
5	2	128-134	131-141	138-150	4	10	102-111	109-121	118-131
5	3	130-136	133-143	140-153	4	11	103-113	111-123	120-134
5	4	132-138	135-145	142-156	5	0	104-115	113-126	122-137
5	5	134-140	137-148	144-160	5	1	106-118	115-129	125-140
5	6	136-142	139-151	146-164	5	2	108-121	118-132	128-143
5	7	138-145	142-154	149-168	5	3	111-124	121-135	131-147
5	8	140-148	145-157	152-172	5	4	114-127	124-138	134-151
5	9	142-151	148-160	155-176	5	5	117-130	127-141	137-155
5	10	144-154	151-163	158-180	5	6	120-133	130-144	140-159
5	11	146-157	154-166	161-184	5	7	123-136	133-147	143-163
6	0	149-160	157-170	164-188	5	8	126-139	136-150	146-167
6	1	152-164	160-174	168-192	5	9	129-142	139-153	149-170
6	2	155-168	164-178	172-197	5	10	132-145	142-156	152-173
6	3	158-172	167-182	176-202	5	11	135-148	145-159	155-176
6	4	162-176	171-187	181-207	6	0	138-151	148-162	158-179

Weight according to frame (ages 25-59) for men wearing indoor clothing weighing 5 lbs., shoes with one-inch heels; for women, indoor clothing weighing 3 lbs., shoes with one-inch heels.
*Reprinted with permission from the Metropolitan Life Insurance Company, New York.

Appendix K: Normal Values and Standards: Fluid Balance

The purpose of the information provided in the Appendix H is to assist the student in answering the workbook's exercises. The lists of normal standards and values is not conclusive. Refer to textbooks for further information if needed.

Normal Fluid Balance in the Adult

<u>Intake</u>
Fluids	1200 mL
Solid food	1000 mL
Water from oxidation	<u>300 mL</u>
	2500 mL

<u>Output</u>
Insensible loss (skin and lungs)	900 mL
In feces	100 mL
Urine	<u>1500 mL</u>
	2500 mL

Commonly Used Fluid Containers and Their Volumes

Water glass	200 ml
Juice glass	120 ml
Cup	180 ml
Soup bowl	
Adult	180 ml
Child	100 ml
Teapot	240 ml
Creamer	
Large	90 ml
Small	30 ml
Water pitcher	1000 ml
Jello, custard dish	100 ml
Ice cream dish	120 ml
Paper cup	
Large	200 ml
Small	120 ml

Appendix L: Medications

The following list of medications is intended to assist the student in answering the exercises in case study #1 and case study #2.

Trade Name: **Alupent**
Generic Name: metaproterenol sulfate
Classification: Beta-adrenergic stimulator, Smooth Muscle Relaxant, Bronchodilator
Uses: Relief of asthma, bronchospasm
Route/Dosage: Oral (Adult): 20 mg every 6 to 8 hours.
Inhalation (Adult): 2 or 3 inhalations, usually not repeated more often than every 3 or 4 hours. Total daily dosage should not exceed 12 inhalations. Each metered dose from inhaler delivers 0.65 metaproterenol.
Side Effects: Nervousness, Tachycardia, Tremor, Nausea

Trade Name: **Benadryl**
Generic Name: diphenhydramine hydrochloride
Classification: Antihistamine
Uses: Relief of allergic conditions; in anaphylaxis as adjunct to epinephrine.
Route/Dosage: Oral, Intramuscular, Intravenous (Adult): 25-50 mg 3 to 4 times a day. Maximum daily dosage 400 mg.
Side Effects: Drowsiness, Dizziness, Headache, Palpitation, dry mouth

Trade Name: **Colace**
Generic Name: docusate sodium
Classficiation: Stool softener, reduces surface tension
Uses: Constipation; and client's who should avoid straining during defecation.
Route/Dosage: Oral (Adults): 50-200 mg/day; adjusted according to individual response
Side Effects: Bitter taste

Generic Name: **Cortisone acetate**
Classification: Anti-inflammatory
Uses: Corticosteroid, glucocorticoid, mineralocorticoid
Route/Dosage: Oral, Intramuscular (Adult): Initial oral dose 25-300 mg daily. Dose reduced by periodic decrements of 10 to 25 mg/day to lowest effective amount.
Side Effects: Sodium and water retention, Increased blood pressure due to retention fluids, Hypokalemia, Suppressed immune response, Increased susceptibility to infection.

Trade Name: **Ecotrin**
Generic Name: acetylsalicylic acid
Classification: Analgesic, Antiinflammatory, Antipyretic
Uses: Long-term aspirin therapy (enteric coated aspirin); antiarthritic; antiplatelet
Route/Dosage: Oral (Adult): Maximum daily dosage 4000 mg divided dosages (e.g., (2) 325 mg tablets every 4 hours).
Side Effects: Gastric irritation and bleeding, Increased bleeding time, Ecchymosis, Ringing in ears

Trade Names: **Ergomar, ergostat**
Generic Name: ergotamine tartrate
Classification: Vasoconstrictor; alpha adrenoreceptor antagonist
Uses: Antimigraine
Route/Dosage: Sublingual (Adult): At start of migraine, sublingual tablet 1-2 mg followed by another 1-2 mg at 30 to 60 minute intervals until attack has abated. Dosage should not exceed 6 mg/24 hours.
Side Effects: Nausea, Vomiting, Diarrhea, Weakness of legs, Numbness, Tingling fingers and toes.

Trade Name: Folex , MTX
Generic Name: methotrexate
Classification: Antineoplastic, Antimetabolic, Folic acid antagonist, Antipsoriatic.
Uses: Principally used in combination regimes to maintain induced remissions in neoplastic diseases.
Route/Dosage: Oral, Intramuscular, Intravenous, Intraarterial, Intrathecal (Adult): Dosage individualized. Orally, 2.5 mg-5.0 mg/day. Treatment course of 5 days.
Side Effects: Oral lesions, GI irritation, Photosensitivity, Hepatic toxicity, Blood dyscrasia

Trade Name: **Metamucil**
Generic Name: psyllium hydrophilic muciloid
Classification: Laxative, Bulk forming
Uses: Constipation
Route/Dosage: Oral (Adult): 1-2 rounded teaspoonfuls one to three times daily; mix in 8 ounces (240 ml) water.
Side Effects: Nausea, Vomiting, Diarrhea with excessive use

Trade Name: **Unipen**
Generic Name: nafcillin
Classification: Antibiotic
Uses: Treatment of infections caused by penicillinase-producing staphylococcus aureus
Route/Dosage: Oral (Adult): 250 mg to 1 Gm every 4 to 6 hours
Intramuscular (Adult): 500 mg every 4 to 6 hours
Intravenous (Adult): 500 mg to 1 Gm every 4 hours
Side Effects: Nausea, Vomiting Diarrhea, Urticaria, Pruritus

Trade Name: **Restoril**
Generic Name: temazepam
Classification: Hypnotic
Uses: Relieve insomnia
Route/Dosage: Oral (Adult): 15 to 30 mg at bedtime
Side Effects: Anorexia, Diarrhea, Drowsiness, Lethargy

Trade Name: **Tylenol #3**
Generic Name: acetaminophen 300 mg with codeine phosphate 30 mg per tablet
Classification: Nonsalicylate analgesic and antipyretic
Combines the analgesic effects of a centrally acting analgesic, codeine, with a peripherally acting analgesic, acetaminophen.
Uses: Relief of mild to moderately severe pain
Route/Dosage: Oral (Adult): one or two tablets every four hours or as required (prn).
Side Effects: Lightheadedness, Dizziness, Sedation, Shortness of breath, Nausea and vomiting, Hepatotoxicity

Trade Name: **Voltaren**
Generic Name: diclofenac sodium
Classification: Nonsteroid, Anti-inflammatory, Analgesic, Antipyretic
Uses: Acute and chronic treatment of rheumatoid arthritis
Route/Dosage: Oral (Adult): Enteric coated tablets; 150-200 mg day in divided doses, 50 mg tid or 75 mg bid
Side Effects: Gastrointestinal toxicity such as; bleeding, ulceration and perforation can occur without warning.

Appendix M: Answers to the Exercises

Exercise A: Identification of Subjective Data P. 25-28

•Pattern #1: Health Perception-Health Management   p. 25

1. "My knuckles are swollen."

2. "...pain...swelling, redness, warmth over knuckles."

3. "I had an infected bunion on my left foot."

4. "I could not taste."

5. "I have felt chills."

6. "...worse attack of arthritis in past 30 years."

7. "I am allergic to methotrexate."

8. "I have felt pain..."

•Pattern #2: Nutritional-Metabolic   p. 25

1. "I sweat a lot."

2. "I feel chilly."

3. "I have lost weight."

4. "I drink 2 juice glasses of water a day."

5. "I have given up using salt."

6. "My mouth is full of sores."

•Pattern #3: Elimination   p. 26

1. "I had blood in my stool several years ago.

2. "I move my bowels every morning."

3. "My stream of urine is slower."

•Pattern #4: Activity-Exercise p. 26

1. "I cannot do anything for myself."

2. "My hands are swollen...hard to move my fingers."

3. "My feet have been puffy."

4. "My blood pressure runs high."

5. "I get tired when I make my breakfast and lunch."

6. "My wife opens all the food containers..."

7. "I hold onto a chair when I walk around."

•Pattern #5: Sleep-Rest   p. 26

1. "My eyes feel tired."

2. "I cannot sleep."

3. "I have no energy."

4. "I am just too tired to talk."

•Pattern #6: Cognitive-Perceptual   p. 27

1. "I hurt in all my joints."

2. "This time, the pain was not relieved with ecotrin."

3. "I rate my pain an 8."

4. "It feels like a knife stabbing each joint."

5. "I cannot taste or smell."

•Pattern #7: Self-Perception/Self-Concept   p. 27

1. "I am not the man I used to be."

2. "My body is bent over and my joints are large."

3. "I am unable to run my photography business."

4. "Please repeat your questions."

5. "I feel badly about my wife working..."

•Pattern #8: Role-Relationship   p. 27

1. "My wife earns the money now...she cares for me."

2. "(Children) help with my business and...house."

3. "My husband needs to accept the fact he cannot work."

•Pattern #9: Sexuality-Reproductive   p. 27

1. "I lost my interest in sex five years ago."

2. "I am too tired and my joints hurt."

•Pattern #10: Coping-Stress Tolerance   p. 28

1. "I pace myself during the day."

2. "I am worried about this infection and joint pain."

3. "...10 years to accept...rheumatoid arthritis."

4. "I perform isometric exercises if I feel tense."

•Pattern #11: Value-Belief   p. 28

1. "My faith in God has helped me."

2. "I enjoy helping other people."

3. "We go to church every Sunday..."

4. "I work in the food pantry and help those in need."

Exercise B: Identification of Subjective Data p. 29-32

•Diagnostic Division # 1: Activity-Rest   p. 29

1. "I am tired at work lately."

2. "I only sleep 2-3 hours."

3. "My eyelids feel very heavy."

4. "I usually sleep 8 hours."

5. "The doctor ordered sleeping medication for me."

6. "I am too tired at work lately."

7. "I walk about 2 miles a day."

•Diagnostic Division #2: Circulation p. 29

1. "My blood pressure runs 120/80."

2. "My heart feels like it is racing."

3. "My head has been pounding the past 2 weeks."

•Diagnostic Division #3: Elimination p. 29

1. "I have a problem with constipation."

2. "...take metamucil everyday...also take colace."

3. "I usually urinate 6 times a day."

•Diagnostic Division #4: Emotional Reactions p. 30

1. "I am concerned about my mastectomy tomorrow."

2. "...will not ruin my chances of wearing a bikini."

3. "This is not fair."

4. "I believe God is punishing me."

5. "I told my husband that I would not go to church..."

6. "I rate my anxiety level a 2."

•Diagnostic Division #5: Food-Fluid p. 30

1. "I feel chilly."

2. "I feel nauseated and too upset to eat today."

3. "I have lost 10 pounds in past 3 weeks."

4. "I eat 3 well balanced meals a day."

5. "I drink 2-3 juice glasses of water a day."

•Diagnostic Division #6: Hygiene p. 30

1. "I shower each day."

2. "I scrub my teeth after every meal."

•Diagnostic Division #7: Neurologic p. 31

1. "I wear glasses to read the newspaper."

2. "My name is Judy Miller...9/3/91...in Urban Hospital."

3. "I have had migraine headaches for the past 20 years."

•Diagnostic Division #8: Pain p. 31

1. "I am having a migraine headache right now."

2. "It is a steady throbbing pain around my left eye."

3. "I rate the intensity a 7 on scale 0-10."

4. "I do not have pain or tenderness in my left breast."

5. "I feel nauseated."

•Diagnostic Division #9:   Relationship Alterations   p. 31

1. "I wish my husband would hurry up and get here."

2. "I am so nervous."

3. "I hope this surgery will not hurt our relationship."

4. "I love my husband and children."

5. "At home, I go for walks to get rid of my anger."

•Diagnostic Division #10:   Safety   p. 31

1. "In 1985, I fell and broke my left wrist and arm."

•Diagnostic Division #11:   Sexuality-Female   p. 32

1. "The doctor told me the tumor was malignant."

2. "I noticed the lump in my left breast..."

3."I have a mammogram...every year for the past 5 years."

4. "We use to have sex once a week."

•Diagnostic Division #12:   Teaching-Learning   p. 32

1. "I drink 5 cups of coffee every day."

2. "I expect to be cured after this surgery."

3. "My...grandmother...my mother died of breast cancer."

4. "My last physical was 2 months ago."

•Diagnostic Division #13:   Ventilation   p. 32

1. "I wheeze when I get asthma."

2. "I never smoke."

3. "My eyes and nose have been itching...."

Exercise C: Identification of Objective Data p. 35-38
•Pattern #1:   Health Perception-Health Management   p. 35

1. Edema right first and second metacarpal phalanges

2. Warmth, redness, edema right metacarpal joints

3. Ulcer left foot crusty yellowish rim. Temp. 101F(R)

4. Lesions throughout oral cavity.

5. Temperature 101F (R). Diaphoretic. Skin warm to touch.

6. No relief symptoms with cortisone injection 8/18/91

7. Methotrexate 2.5 mg/qd x 5 days. Discontinued 8/18/91

8. Facial grimacing; moaning upon joint movement.

•Pattern #2:   Nutritional-Metabolic   p. 35

1. Skin turgor: shape returned in 15 seconds

2. Temperature 101F (R). Skin hot to touch. Diaphoretic.

3. Weight loss 10 lbs. past 6 months.

4. 24 hour oral fluid intake 930cc

5. Low sodium 2g pureed diet ordered by physician.

6. Lesions throughout buccal mucosa.

•Pattern #3:   Elimination   p. 36

1. 9/3/91 No melena in stool specimen.

2. Abdomen nondistended, nontender.

3. Internist noted decrease in force urine stream

•Pattern #4:   Activity-Exercise   p. 36

1. 70 degree elbow flexion

2. Weak hand grasp. Swelling metacarpal phalange joints.

3. Both ankles 2+ edema

4. BP 150/90

5. Sat down twice enroute bathroom 10 ft. from bed.

6. Weak hand grasp.

7. Unsteady gait and balance when walking.

•Pattern #5:   Sleep-Rest   p. 36

1. Ptosis of eyelids

2. Dark circles under eyes. Ptosis eyelids.

3. Yawning throughout interview.

4. Mispronounces words.

•Pattern #6:   Cognitive-Perceptual   p. 37

1. Facial grimacing.

2. Ecotrin 325 mg, 2 tablets/ 4 times qd

3. Facial grimacing/moaning when joints tested for ROM

4. Facial grimacing and moaning upon movement joint

5. Inability to identify smell of alcohol or taste coffee

•Pattern #7:   Self-Perception/Self-Concept   p. 37

1. Spoke in halting low voice.

2. Stooped posture with little body movement.

3. Behavior rated 2.

4. Easily distracted. Interview questions repeated.

5. Looked at floor or wall during interview.

•Pattern #8:   Role-Relationship   p. 37

1. Wife holding client's hand during interview.

2. Social worker noted children assist with business.

3. Wife and client observed in problem solving situation.

•Pattern #9:   Sexuality-Reproductive   p. 37

1. Mumbling responses to questions

2. No eye contact with interviewer.

•Pattern #10:   Coping-Stress Tolerance   p. 38

1. Paces energy level.

2. Facial muscles taut.

3. No wringing hands.Rated anxiety level 2 on scale 0-5.

4. Demonstrated isometric exercises.

•Pattern #11:   Value-Belief   p. 38

1. Bible on bedside stand.

2. Many get-well cards posted on the wall.

3. Chaplain's pamphlet lying on bedside stand.

4. Smiled when talking about helping others.

Exercise D: Identification of Objective Data   p. 39-42
•Division #1:   Activity-Rest   p. 39

1. Slight hand tremor.

2. Dark circles under eyes.

3. Ptosis of eyelids.

4. Decreased attention span.

5. Temazapam 30 mg Tab 1 (o) qhs prn

6. Yawning during interview. Slouched posture.

7. Firm muscle tone. No dyspnea upon exertion.

•Division #2:   Circulation   p. 39

1. Actual blood pressure 150/80 mm Hg

2. Pulse rate 90.

3. Rubbing forehead over left eye. BP 150/80. P 90.

•Division #3:   Elimination   p. 39

1. Hard, formed, brown colored stool.

2. Abdomen moderately distended. Colace 100 mgm qd prn.

3. Specific gravity 1.025. Urine straw colored, clear.

•Division #4: Emotional Reactions   p. 40

1. Facial muscles taut.

2. Speaking in a loud abrupt voice.

3. Eyes darting around the room.

4. Face flushed.

5. Constantly talking.

6. Face flushed. Facial muscles taut. BP 150/80. P 90.R 24

•Division #5: Food-Fluid   p. 40

1. Skin warm to touch.

2. Ate 25% food on lunch tray.

3. Actual weight 110 pounds. 5 feet 6 inches.

4. Daily 3 meals not balanced with basic 4 food groups.

5. Skin turgor: Shape returned in 10 seconds.

•Division #6: Hygiene   p. 40

1. Skin clean.

2. No plaque present. No dentures/plate.32 permanent teeth

•Division #7: Neurologic   p. 40

1. Reads newsprint with glasses.

2. Oriented to time, place and person

3. Physician noted 20 year history treatment migraine.

•Division #8: Pain   p. 41

1. Facial grimacing.

2. Rubbing forehead over left eye.

3. Palpable neck and shoulder muscles.

4. Hard, irregular, poorly delineated, nonmobile lump.

5. Skin pale, perspiring

•Division #9: Relationship Alterations   p. 41

1. Husband not present.

2. Wringing hands. Pacing floor.

3. Began crying.

4. Smiled when talking about husband and child.

5. Began pacing floor. Wringing hands.

•Division #10: Safety   p. 41

1. Wrist 80-90 degree flexion and extension.

•Division #11: Sexuality-Female p. 41

1. Left breast biopsy positive primary tumor stage T1.

2. Demonstrated correct self-examination breast

3. Diagnostic studies reflect yearly mammogram 1986-1991.

4. Frown on face when discussing sexual relationship.

•Division #12: Teaching-Learning p. 42

1. Drank 500-750 mg caffeine in coffee per day.

2. Wringing hands.

3. Genogram reflects family history breast cancer.

4. Chart reflects yearly physical 1986-1991.

•Division #13: Ventilation p. 42

1. Minimal wheezing upon expiration.

2. Chest x-ray negative. No emphysema/SOB.

3. Nasal turbinates, pale, edematous, watery drainage.

Exercise E: Data Validation p. 45-51

•Pattern #1: Health Perception/Management p. 45

1. Client Value:

SD: "My knuckles are swollen."

OD: Edema right first and second metacarpal phalanges

Normal Value: No edema metacarpal joints

2. Client Value:

SD: "...pain...swelling,redness, warmth over knuckles

OD: Warmth, redness, edema right metacarpal joints

Normal Value: No signs or symptoms of inflammation

3. Client Value:

SD: "I had an infected bunion on my left foot."

OD: Ulcer left foot crusty yellowish rim. Temp.101F(R)

Normal Value: No crusting, signs or symptoms infection

4. Client Value:

SD: "I could not taste."

OD: Lesions throughout oral cavity.

Normal Value: Sense of taste.Numerous taste buds tongue

5. Client Value:

SD: "I felt chills."

OD: Temperature 101 F (R).Diaphoretic. Skin warm touch

Normal Value: Temperature for age 98.6 F(o)/99.6 F(R)

6. Client Value:

SD: "...worse attack of arthritis in past 30 years."

OD: No relief symptoms with cortisone 8/18/91

Normal Value: Anti-inflammatory action cortisone

7. Client Value:

SD: "I am allergic to methotrexate."

OD: 8/12/91 Methotrexate 2.5 mg/qd x5days. D/C 8/18/91

Normal Value: No allergic reaction to methotrexate

8. Client Value:

SD: "I have felt pain..."

OD: Facial grimacing; moaning upon joint movement.

Normal Value: Full range of motion without joint pain

•Pattern #2: Nutritional-Metabolic p. 46

1. Client Value:

SD: "I sweat a lot."

OD: Skin turgor: Shape returned in 15 seconds

Normal Value: Prompt return of skin to normal position

2. Client Value:

SD: "I feel chilly."

OD: Temp. 101F (R). Skin hot to touch. Diaphoretic

Normal Value: No temperature.Skin warm.No diaphoresis

3. Client Value:

SD: "I have lost weight."

OD: Weight loss 10 lbs. past 6 months.

Normal Value: Maintain normal weight.

4. Client Value:

SD: "I drink 2 juice glasses of water a day."

OD: 24 hour oral fluid intake 930cc

Normal Value: 1200cc oral/2500cc total fluid intake/24h

5. Client Value:

SD: "I have given up using salt."

OD: Low sodium, 2 g pureed diet ordered by physician

Normal Value: 1100-3300mg sodium/qd

6. Client Value:

SD: "My mouth is full of sores."

OD: Lesions throughout buccal mucosa.

Normal Value: No lesions buccal mucosa.

•Pattern #3: Elimination   p. 46

1. Client Value:

SD: "I had blood in my stool several years ago."

OD: 9/3/91 No melena

Normal Value: No melena

2. Client Value:

SD: "I move my bowels every morning."

OD: Abdomen nondistended, nontender

Normal Value: Nondistended, nontender abdomen.

3. Client Value:

SD: "My stream of urine is slower."

OD: Internist noticed decrease in force urine stream

Normal Value: Ability detrusor muscles to contract

•Pattern #4: Activity-Exercise   p. 47

1. Client Value:

SD: "I cannot do anything for myself."

OD: 70 degrees elbow flexion

Normal Value: 150 degrees elbow flexion

2. Client Value:

SD: "My hands are swollen...hard to move my fingers"

OD: Weak hand grasp.Swelling metacarpal phalange joints

Normal Value: No swelling joints. Ability grasp firmly.

3. Client Value:

SD: "My feet have been puffy."

OD: Both ankles 2+ edema

Normal Value: No edema present.

4. Client Value:

SD: "My blood pressure runs high."

OD: BP 140/70

Normal Value: BP 120/80 age

5. Client Value:

SD: "I get tired when I make my breakfast and lunch."

OD: Sat down twice enroute bathroom 10 ft. from bed.

Normal Value: Ability perform activities daily living

6. Client Value:

SD: "My wife opens all the food containers..."

OD: Weak hand grasp.

Normal Value: Firm hand grasp. Ability perform ADL.

7. Client Value:

SD: "I hold onto a chair when I walk around."

OD: Unsteady gait and balance when walking.

Normal Value: Steady gait and balance when walking.

•Pattern #5:   Sleep-Rest   p. 48

1. Client Value:

SD: "My eyes feel tired."

OD: Ptosis of eyelids

Normal Value: No ptosis (drooping) of eyelids

2. Client Value:

SD: "I cannot sleep."

OD: Dark circles under eyes. Ptosis eyelids

Normal Value: No dark circles under eyes.No ptosis lids

3. Client Value:

SD: "I have no energy."

OD: Yawning throughout interview.

Normal Value: Sufficient energy to perform ADL

4. Client Value:

SD: "I am just too tired to talk."

OD: Mispronounces words.

Normal Value: Ability communicate clearly

•Pattern #6:   Cognitive-Perceptual   p. 48

1. Client Value:

SD: "I hurt in all my joints."

OD: Facial grimacing

Normal Value: No joint pain

2. Client Value:

SD: "...the pain was not relieved with ecotrin."

OD: Order for Ecotrin 325 mg, 2 tablets 4 times qd.

Normal Value: Ecotrin 4000 mg (o) divided doses

3. Client Value:

SD: "I rate my pain an 8."

OD: Facial grimacing/moaning joints tested for ROM

Normal Value: Full ROM without pain

4. Client Value:

SD: "It feels like a knife stabbing each joint."

OD: Facial grimacing and moaning upon movement joint

Normal Value: Full ROM without pain

5. Client Value:

SD: "I cannot taste or smell."

OD: Inability identify smell alcohol and taste coffee

Normal Value: Sense of taste and smell intact

•Pattern #7: Self-Perception/Concept   p. 49

1. Client Value:

SD: "I am not the man I should be."

OD: Spoke in halting, low voice.

Normal Value: Feelings of self-worth

2. Client Value:

SD: "My body is bent over and my joints are large."

OD: Stooped posture with little body movement.

Normal Value: Erect posture. No enlarged joints.

3. Client Value:

SD: "I am unable to run my photography business."

OD: Behavior rated 2.

Normal Value: Behavior (1) passive to (5) assertive

4. Client Value:

SD: "Please repeat your questions."

OD: Easily distracted. Interview questions repeated.

Normal Value: Ability concentrate on task at hand.

5. Client Value:

SD: "I feel badly about my wife working..."

OD: Looked at floor or wall during interview.

Normal Value: Positive feelings of human value

•Pattern #8: Role-Relationship p. 49

1. Client Value:

SD: "My wife the money now...she cares for me."

OD: Wife holding client's hand

Normal Value: Caring relationship

2. Client Value:

SD: "(Children) help with my business and ...house."

OD: Social worker noted children assist with business

Normal Value: Supportive family relationships

3. Client Value:

SD: "My husband needs accept the fact...cannot work."

OD: Wife/client observed in problem solving situation

Normal Value: Use cognitive skills deal with stressor

•Pattern #9: Sexuality-Reproductive p. 50

1. Client Value:

SD: "I never asked my wife if it bothered her."

OD: Mumbling responses to questions.

Normal Value: Ability to express self to loved ones

2. Client Value:

SD: "I am too tired and my joint hurt."

OD: No eye contact with interviewer.

Normal Value: Ability to express self to interviewer.

•Pattern #10: Coping-Stress Tolerance p. 50

1. Client Value:

SD: "I pace myself during the day."

OD: Paces energy level

Normal Value: Time management to conserve energy

2. Client Value:

SD: "I am worried about this infection and joint pain."

OD: Facial muscles taut.

Normal Value: Toned facial muscles.Ability express fears

3. Client Value:

SD: "...10 years accept...rheumatoid arthritis."

OD:No wringing hands.Rated anxiety level 2 scale 0-5

Normal Value: Recognition limitations/ impact disease

4. Client Value:

SD: "I perform isometric exercises if I feel tense."

OD: Demonstrated isometric exercises.

Normal Value: Isometric exercise increase strength

•Pattern #11: Value-Belief p. 51

1. Client Value:

SD: "My faith in God has helped me."

OD: Bible on bedside stand.

Normal Value: Belief system provides meaning to life

2. Client Value:

SD: "I enjoy helping other people."

OD: Many get-well cards posted on the wall.

Normal Value: Social support system for times of stress

3. Client Value:

SD: "We go to church every Sunday..."

OD: Chaplain's pamphlet lying on bedside stand.

Normal Value: Belief system provides support

4. Client Value:

SD: "I work in the food pantry...help those in need."

OD: Smiled when talking about helping others.

Normal Value: Helping others increases self-worth

Exercise F: Data Validation p. 53-59

•Division #1: Activity-Rest p. 53

1. Client Value:

SD: "I am tired at work lately."

OD: Slight hand tremor

Normal Value: No hand tremor

2. Client Value:

SD: "I sleep only 2-3 hours."

OD: Dark circles under eyes.

Normal Value: No dark circles. 6-7 hours sleep/night.

3. Client Value:

SD: "My eyelids feel very heavy."

OD: Ptosis of eyelids.

Normal Value: No ptosis.

4. Client Value:

SD: "I usually sleep 8 hours."

OD: Decreased attention span.

Normal Value: Ability to concentrate on task at hand.

5. Client Value:

SD: "The doctor ordered sleeping medication for me."

OD: Temazapam 30 mg Tab 1 (o) qhs prn

Normal Value: Ability to sleep without sedatives.

6. Client Value:

SD: "I am too tired at work lately."

OD: Yawning during interview. Slouched posture.

Normal Value: No yawning. Posture erect.

7. Client Value:

SD: "walk about 2 miles a day."

OD: Firm muscle tone. No dyspnea upon exertion.

Normal Value: Firm muscle tone.No dyspnea upon exertion

•Division #2: Circulation   p. 54

1. Client Value:

SD: "My usual blood pressure is 120/80."

OD: Actual BP 150/80 mm Hg

Normal Value: 120/80 mm Hg

2. Client Value:

SD: "My heart feels like it is racing."

OD: Pulse rate 90 at rest.

Normal Value: Average pulse for age 70-75.

3. Client Value:

SD: "My head has been pounding the past 2 weeks."

OD: Rubbing forehead over left eye. BP 150/80. P 90

Normal Value: No pounding. BP 120/80. P 70-75.

•Division #3: Elimination   p. 54

1. Client Value:

SD: "I have a problem with constipation."

OD: Hard, formed, brown colored stool

Normal Value: Formed, moist stool

2. Client Value:

SD: "..take metamucil everyday...take colace once day.

OD: Abdomen moderately distended.Colace 100 mg(o)qd prn

Normal Value: Regular bowel movements without laxatives

3. Client Value:

SD: "I usually urinate six times during the day."

OD: Specific gravity urine 1.025;straw colored,clear

Normal Value: Sp.grav.1.003-1.030.Clear, star colored

•Division #4: Emotional Reactions   p. 54

1. Client Value:

SD: "I am concerned about my mastectomy tomorrow."

OD: Facial muscles taut

Normal Value: Toned, not taut facial muscles

2. Client Value:

SD: "I hope I can wear a bikini after this surgery."

OD: Speaking in loud abrupt. Constantly talking.

Normal Value: Support system helps reduce stress level

3. Client Value:

SD: "This is not fair."

OD: Eyes darting around room.

Normal Value: Demonstrates effective coping skills.

4. Client Value:

SD: "I believe God is punishing me."

OD: Face flushed. Facial muscles taut.

Normal Value: Reality orientation to the cause of problem.

5. Client Value:

SD: "I told my husband...I would not go church anymore"

OD: Constantly talking.

Normal Value: Problem solving. No transference problem.

6. Client Value:

SD: "I rate my anxiety level a 2."

OD: Face flushed/muscles taut.BP 150/80.P 90.R 24

Normal Value: Rates anxiety level 0. Free undue anxiety.

•Division #5:   Food-Fluid   p. 55
1. Client Value:

SD: "I feel chilly."

OD: Skin cool to touch

Normal Value: Skin warm to touch

2. Client Value:

SD: "I feel nauseated and too upset to eat today."

OD: Ate 25% food on lunch tray.

Normal Value: Recommended nutrients consumed qd

3. Client Value:

SD: "I have lost 10 pounds in past 3 weeks."

OD: Actual weight 110 pounds; 5'6".. Small frame.

Normal Value: Weight 136-142 lbs./5'6"/small frame

4. Client Value:

SD: "I eat 3 well-balanced meals a day."

OD: Daily dietary intake lacked basic 4 food groups.

Normal Value: Recommended amount nutrients consumed qd

5. Client Value:

SD: "I drink 2-3 juice glasses of water a day."

OD: Skin turgor: shape returned in 10 seconds.

Normal Value: 1200 cc intake qd. Immediate return skin.

•Division #6:   Hygiene   p. 56
1. Client Value:

SD: "I shower every day."

OD: Skin clean

Normal Value: Daily hygiene

2. Client Value:

SD: "I scrub my teeth after every meal."

OD: 32 permanent teeth. No plaque. No dentures/plate

Normal Value: 32 permanent teeth.No plaque/dentures

•Division #7:   Neurologic   p. 56
1. Client Value:

SD: "I wear glasses at work to read the fine print."

OD: Reads newsprint with glasses

Normal Value: Read newsprint without glasses

2. Client Value:

SD: "...Judy Smith...9/3/91...Urban Hospital..."

OD: Oriented to time, place and person.

Normal Value: Oriented to time, place and person.

3. Client Value:

SD: "...migraine headaches for the past 20 years."

OD: Physician's note stated 20 year treatment migraine.

Normal Value: No migraine headaches.

•Division #8: Pain p. 56

1. Client Value:

SD: "I am having a migraine headache right now."

OD: Facial grimacing

Normal Value: No headaches

2. Client Value:

SD: "It is a steady throbbing pain over my left eye."

OD: Rubbing forehead over left eye.Lights off in room.

Normal Value: No pain over left eye.

3. Client Value:

SD: "I rate the intensity a 7 on scale of 1-10."

OD: Palpable neck and shoulder muscles.

Normal Value: 0 intensity. Normal neck/shoulder muscles

4. Client Value:

SD: "I do not have pain/tenderness in...left breast."

OD: Hard, irregular, poorly delineated, nonmobile lump

Normal Value: Breast cancer painless 90% cases

5. Client Value:

SD: "...I feel nauseated."

OD: Skin pale, perspiring.

Normal Value: Pigmentation ranges from ivory/deep brown, skin moist. No nausea.

•Division #9: Relationship Alterations p.57

1. Client Value:

SD: "I wish my husband would hurry up and get here."

OD: Husband not present at admission interview.

Normal Value: Significant other provides support system

2. Client Value:

SD: "I am so nervous."

OD: Wringing hands. Pacing floor.

Normal Value: Effective coping skills relieve anxiety

3. Client Value:

SD: "I hope this surgery...not hurt our relationship"

OD: Began crying.

Normal Value: Family assist in working through emotions

4. Client Value:

SD: "I love my husband and children."

OD: Smiled when talking about husband and children.

Normal Value: Share love and belonging with others

5. Client Value:

SD: "At home, I go for walks to get rid of my anger."

OD: Began pacing floor. Wringing hands.

Normal Value: Effective coping skills relieve anxiety

•Division #10:   Safety   p. 58

1. Client Value:

SD: "In 1985, I fell and broke my left wrist."

OD: Wrist 80-90 degree flexion and extension

Normal Value: Wrist 80-90 degree flexion/extension

•Division #11:   Sexuality-Female   p. 58

1. Client Value:

SD: "The doctor told me the tumor was malignant."

OD: Breast biopsy positive for primary tumor stage T1.

Normal Value: No breast tumor. Negative biopsy results

2. Client Value:

SD: "I noticed the lump..during my monthly self exam"

OD: Demonstrated correct self-breast examination.

Normal Value: Monthly self-breast exam regular time

3. Client Value:

SD: "I had a mammogram...every year past 5 years."

OD: Diagnostic studies...yearly mammogram 1986-1991

Normal Value: Yearly mammogram after age 50.

4. Client Value:

SD: "We use to have sex once a week."

OD: Frown on face when discussing sexual relations.

Normal Value: Cognitive knowledge re: human sexuality

•**Division #12: Teaching-Learning p. 58**
1. Client Value:

SD: "I drink 5 cups of coffee every day."

OD: Drank 500-750 mg caffeine per day.

Normal Value: 100-150 mg caffeine/qd;100-150mg c. coffee

2. Client Value:

SD: "I expect to be cured after the surgery."

OD: Wringing hands.

Normal Value: Realistic expectations from surgery.

3. Client Value:

SD: "My mother and grandmother died of breast cancer..."

OD: Genogram reflects family history breast cancer.

Normal Value:Presence risk factors predisposes disease

4. Client Value:

SD: "My last physical exam was 2 months ago."

OD: Chart reflects yearly physical exams 1986-1991.

Normal Value: Yearly examinations provide baseline data

•**Division #13: Ventilation p. 59**
1. Client Value:

SD: "I wheeze when I get asthma."

OD: Minimal wheezing upon expiration.

Normal Value: Lungs clear auscultation. No allergies

2. Client Value:

SD: "I never smoke."

OD: Chest x-ray negative. No emphysema/SOB.

Normal Value: Chest x-ray negative. No emphysema/SOB

3. Client Value:

SD: "My eyes and nose have been itchy."

OD: Nasal turbinates pale, edematous. Lacrimation.

Normal Value: No edema nasal turbinates.No tearing eyes

Exercise G: Identification of Dysfunctional Health Patterns, p. 63-64

•Pattern #1:   Health Perception-Health Management   p. 63

Dysfunctional   YES X   NO __
Rationale: Subjective data (e.g., increase in joint pain) and objective data (e.g., elevated WBC) demonstrated the signs and symptoms of inflammation and infection, resulting in exacerbation of the rheumatoid arthritis.

•Pattern #2:   Nutritional-Metabolic   p. 63

Dysfunctional   YES X_   NO __
Rationale: Demonstrated decreased skin turgor with fluid intake less than normal 1200cc/24h. Lesions through out buccal mucosa interfered with taste sensation and mastication of food.

•Pattern #3:   Elimination   p. 63

Dysfunctional   YES __   NO X
Rationale: 9/3/91 stool specimen negative for melena. Decrease in force urine. Majority values within normal limits.

•Pattern #4:   Activity-Exercise   p. 63

Dysfunctional   YES X   NO __
Rationale: Subjective data (e.g., lack of energy) and objective data (e.g., unsteady gait, limited ROM, and enlargement of joints) validate client's inability to perform ADL without assistance. Elevated blood pressure and 2+ edema both feet may indicate cardiovascular problem.

•Pattern #5:   Sleep-Rest   p. 63

Dysfunctional   YES X_   NO __
Rationale: Verbal expressions of fatigue and inability to sleep. Change from optimal adult sleep pattern of 7-8 hours for age resulting in lack of energy to perform ADL.

•Pattern #6:   Cognitive-Perceptual   p. 63

Dysfunctional   YES X   NO __
Rationale: Verbalized increased pain in all joints. Pain elicited upon movement of joints. Perceived no relief with pain medication. Present pain management ineffective in alleviating pain. Diminished sense of taste and smell.

•Pattern #7:   Self-Perception/Self-Concept   p. 64

Dysfunctional   YES X_   NO __
Rationale: Low self-esteem due to decrease in physical abilities, changes in body function and appearance. Inability to manage own business. Decreased attention span; behavior passive.

•Pattern #8:   Role-Relationship   p. 64

Dysfunctional   YES __   NO X
Rationale: Wife earns sufficient income to meet families financial needs. Client demonstrated ability to verbalize feelings regarding the change in the roles of family members. Wife and children provide family support system. Majority of findings within normal limits (WNL).

•Pattern #9:   Sexuality-Reproductive   p. 64

Dysfunctional   YES X_   NO __
Rationale: Inability to verbalize perceived changes in sexuality pattern with partner. Progression of the client's disease process has prevented the continuation of previous sexual expressions. No evidence of counseling in this area.

•Pattern #10:   Coping-Stress Tolerance   p. 64

Dysfunctional   YES __   NO X
Rationale: Ability to identify fears and concerns. Recognizes limitations. Implemented strategies to reduce stress. Family support system in place. Majority of findings within normal limits.

•Pattern #11: Value-Belief   p. 64

Dysfunctional   YES __   NO X

Rationale: Practiced beliefs and values that also served as a coping strategy. Ability to extend self to others in need. Social support system in place. Wife, husband and children share common beliefs and values. Majority findings within normal limits.

Exercise H: Identification of Dysfunctional Diagnostic Divisions p. 65-66

•Division #1: Activity-Rest   p. 65

Dysfunctional   YES X   NO __

Rationale: Verbalized changes in sleeping habit from optimal adult sleep pattern of 7-8 hours for age. Slept 2-3 hours per night past 2 months. Subjective data (e.g., verbal expressions of fatigue) and objective data (e.g., dark circles under eyes) failed to meet accepted normal standards and values.

•Division #2: Circulation   p. 65

Dysfunctional   YES X   NO X

Rationale: Changes noted from client's baseline values and accepted normal values. Elevated blood pressure (150/80), increased pulse rate (90) and increased respirations (24). Verbalized sensation of head pounding. Values failed to meet accepted normal standards and values.

•Division #3: Elimination   p. 65

Dysfunctional   YES X   NO __

Rationale: Client verbalized changes in regularity of bowel elimination habits (e.g., constipation for the past 2 months). Insufficient roughage in diet. Stool softeners ineffective in remedying problem.

•Division #4: Emotional Reactions   p. 65

Dysfunctional   YES X   NO __

Rationale: Verbalized increase in anxiety level (e.g., rated anxiety level a 2). Fear mastectomy will change her body image and relationship with husband. Ineffective individual and family coping skills demonstrated.

•Division #5: Food-Fluid   p. 65

Dysfunctional   YES X   NO __

Rationale: Verbalized deviation from normal daily intake of food due to nausea. Weight 20% below ideal for height and frame. Weight loss indicated insufficient intake of nutrients to meet metabolic needs. Demonstrated decreased skin turgor with fluid intake less than normal 1200cc/24h

•Division #6: Hygiene   p. 65

Dysfunctional   YES __   NO X

Rationale: Ability to meet daily hygiene needs. Values within normal limits.

•Division #7: Neurologic   p. 56

Dysfunctional   YES __   NO X

Rationale: Majority of data within normal limits. Migraine headaches addressed under the diagnostic division: pain.

•Division #8: Pain   p. 56

Dysfunctional   YES X   NO __

Rationale: Subjective data (e.g., nausea, rated pain a 7 on scale 0-10) and objective data (e.g., facial grimacing, rubbing forehead over left eye) provided evidence that the pain management was ineffective in alleviating the migraine headaches.

•Division #9: Relationship Alterations   p. 57

Dysfunctional   YES X   NO X

Rationale: Proposed change in body (mastectomy) caused a threat to client's self-concept and self-esteem. Husband not present. Lack of support from significant other increased client's anxiety level. Verbalized fear of mastectomy affecting relationship with husband. Lack of effective individual and family coping skills.

•**Division #10:** **Safety** **p. 58**

Dysfunctional   YES __   NO X

Rationale: Majority clustered data within normal limits. Hay fever discussed under diagnostic division: Ventilation

•**Division #11:** **Sexuality** **p. 58**

Dysfunctional   YES X   NO __

Rationale: Verbalized fear of husband's possibledissatisfaction with sexual relations due to mastectomy. Expressed perceived threat to sexual role. Inability of partners to discuss openly their feelings regarding the forthcoming mastectomy. No problem solving evident.

•**Division #12:** **Teaching-Learning** **p. 58**

Dysfunctional   YES X   NO __

Rationale: Verbalized unrealistic expectations of surgery. Familial history of breast cancer. Intake of caffeine per day exceeded normal values (e.g., drank 500-750mg caffeine in her coffee per day). Excessive ingestion of caffeine may cause insomnia, restlessness, nausea and tachycardia.

•**Division #13:** **Ventilation** **p. 59**

Dysfunctional   YES __   NO X

Rationale: History of hay fever and asthma. Inability to maintain clear airway at all times due to edema of nasal mucosa. Minimal wheezing sounds on expiration.

Exercise I: Identification of Nursing Diagnoses p. 71-72

1. Nursing Diagnosis: Altered Protection

    Etiology (related to): immunosuppression

    Defining Characteristics (as evidenced by): WBC 11,000; culture positive staphylococcus aureus; heat, redness and swelling joints.

2. Nursing Diagnosis: Alteration in Oral Mucous Membrane

    Etiology (related to): drug reaction

    Defining Characteristics (as evidenced by): presence buccal lesions, decreased sense of taste, oral pain.

3. Nursing Diagnosis: Impaired Physical Mobility: Level I

    Etiology (related to): uncompensated musculoskeletal impairment

    Defining Characteristics (as evidenced by):unsteady gait, limited range of motion, decreased muscle strength.

4. Nursing Diagnosis: Sleep Pattern Disturbance

    Etiology (related to): physical discomfort

    Defining Characteristics (as evidenced by): dark circles under eyes, ptosis of eyelids, verbalized feelings of fatigue.

5. Nursing Diagnosis: Pain

    Etiology (related to): chronic physical disability

    Defining Characteristics (as evidenced by) : facial grimacing, verbalization of pain upon movement of joints; rated pain 8 on scale 0-10.

6. Nursing Diagnosis: Self-Esteem Disturbance

    Etiology (related to): loss of significant role

    Defining Characteristics (as evidenced by) : decrease in physical abilities stooped posture, verbalized changes in body appearance.

7. Nursing Diagnosis: Altered Sexuality Patterns

    Etiology (related to): change in body functions

    Defining Characteristics (as evidenced by): limitation and pain of physical movement, inability discuss perceived changes with wife.

Exercise J: Formulating a Nursing Diagnostic Statement p. 73-75

1. Nursing Diagnosis: Sleep-Pattern Disturbance

    Etiology (related to): personal stress

    Defining Characteristics (as evidenced by): ptosis of eyelids, dark circles under eyes, verbalized inability to sleep.

2. Nursing Diagnosis: Constipation

    Etiology (related to): low roughage diet and fluid intake

    Defining Characteristics (as evidenced by): hard formed stools, use laxatives, fluid intake less normal 1200cc/ 24h.

3. Nursing Diagnosis: Body Image Disturbance

    Etiology (related to): perceived threat to self concept

    Defining Characteristics (as evidenced by): verbalized increase in anxiety level, change in relationship with husband, fear appearing less sexually attractive to husband.

4. Nursing Diagnosis: Fluid Volume Deficit

    Etiology (related to): deviation from normal fluid intake

    Defining Characteristics (as evidenced by): intake below normal 1200/qd, decreased skin turgor, Hct 50%

5. Nursing Diagnosis: Pain

    Etiology (related to): physiological injuring agent

    Defining Characteristics (as evidenced by): verbalized steady throbbing pain over left eye; rated pain 7 on scale 0-10; increased vital signs.

6. Nursing Diagnosis: Altered Family Processes

    Etiology (related to): situational crisis

    Defining Characteristics (as evidenced by): lack of support from husband, husband's inability to express feelings, client's verbal expressions of anxiety.

7. Nursing Diagnosis: Altered Sexual Patterns

    Etiology (related to): change in body function

    Defining Characteristics (as evidenced by): perceived threat sexual role, fear of husband's dissatisfaction with

             client's body   change, changes in husband's sexual behavior.

8. Nursing Diagnosis: Knowledge Deficit-Therapeutic Regime

    Etiology (related to): misinterpretation therapeutic interventions

    Defining Characteristics (as evidenced by) :unrealistic expectations surgery results; excessive consumption

             of stimulant caffeine; unrealistic expectations of postoperative

             recovery period

9. Nursing Diagnosis: Ineffective Airway Clearance

    Etiology (related to): excess thick secretions

    Defining Characteristics (as evidenced by): nasal mucosa edematous, nasal discharge, verbalized pruritus of

             eyes, eyes tearing, wheezing sounds on expiration, respirations

             24, diaphoretic.

Exercise K: Ranking Nursing Diagnoses p. 81

Nursing Diagnoses	Maslow's Needs	Ranking
1. Altered Protection	Safety	High
2. Pain	Physiological	High
3. Altered Oral Mucous Membrane	Physiological	Medium
4. Impaired Physical Mobility	Physiological	Medium
5. Sleep-Pattern Disturbance	Physiological	Medium
6. Self-Esteem Disturbance	Self esteem	Low
7. Altered Sexuality Patterns	Love/Belonging	Low

Exercise L: Ranking Nursing Diagnoses p. 82

Nursing Diagnoses	Maslow's Needs	Ranking
1. Ineffective Airway Clearance	Physiological	High
2. Fluid Volume Deficit	Physiological	High
3. Pain	Physiological	High
4. Knowledge Deficit	Safety	Medium
5. Altered Family Processes	Love/Belonging	Medium
6. Body Image Disturbance	Love/Belonging	Medium
7. Sleep Pattern Disturbance	Physiological	Medium
8. Constipation	Physiological	Medium
9. Altered Sexual Patterns	Love/Belonging	Low

Exercise M: Formulating Outcome Criteria p. 87-88

•1. Outcome Criteria

Subject: Client

Measurable Verb: will demonstrate

Outcome: changing of dressing on left bunion

Criteria: accurately

Target Time: by 9/20/91

•2. Outcome Criteria

Subject: Client

Measurable Verb: will practice

Outcome: slow rhythmic breathing

Criteria: independently before pain rating reaches 4.

Target Time: by day 9/4/91.

•3. Outcome Criteria

Subject: Client

Measurable verb: will rinse

Outcome: buccal mucosa, tongue, gums with saline

Criteria: after each meal and at bedtime

Target Time: by day 9/5/91.

•4. Outcome Criteria

Subject: Client

Measurable Verb: will walk

Outcome: with a walker

Criteria: safely walk 20 feet 4 times a day

Target Time: 9/14/91

Exercise N: Formulating Outcome Criteria p. 89-90

•1. Outcome Criteria

Subject: Client

Measurable Verb: will deep breath and cough

Outcome: using abdominal and accessory muscles

Criteria: 5 minutes every one hour while awake

Target Time: by 9/5/91

•2. Outcome Criteria

Subject: Client

Measurable Verb: will demonstrate

Outcome: fluid and electrolyte balance

Criteria: within normal limits

Target Time: during the perioperative period

•3. Outcome Criteria

Subject: Client

Measurable Verb: will practice

Outcome: guided imagery and rhythmic breathing

Criteria: onset migraine/q1h migraine rated below 4

Target Time: 9/4/91

•4. Outcome Criteria

Subject: Client and husband

Measurable Verb: will describe

Outcome: postoperative outcomes, possible complications, and discharge planning

Criteria: realistically and accurately

Target Time: before scheduled surgery

Exercise O: Writing Nursing Orders   p. 93-94

•1. Nursing Order

Measurable Verb: Teach

Subject: client and wife

Outcome: aseptic dressing change on bunion

Target Time: by 9/5/91

Signature: Cyndie Smith, RN

•2. Nursing Order

Measurable Verb: Teach

Subject: client

Outcome: pain reduction through rhythmic breathing

Target Time: 9/3/91

Signature: Cyndie Smith, RN

•3. Nursing Order

Measurable Verb: Demonstrate

Subject: to client

Outcome: medical asepsis techniques used to cleanse mouth

Target Time: 9/3/91

Signature: Cyndie Smith, RN

•4. Nursing order

Measurable verb: Demonstrate

Subject: to client and wife

Outcome: safe ambulating techniques with a walker

Target time: by 9/5/91

Signature: Cyndie Smith, RN

Exercise P: Writing Nursing Orders   p. 95-96

1. Nursing Order

Measurable Verb: Explain and demonstrate

Subject: to client

Outcome: therapeutic effects deep breathing/coughing q1h

Target Time: 9/3/91

Signature: Kathy Mayer, RN

•2. Nursing Order

Measurable Verb: Monitor

Subject: client's

Outcome: intake & output;blood chemistry/hematology values for compliance with normal values

Target Time: during perioperative period

Signature: Kathy Mayer, RN

•3. Nursing Order

Measurable Verb: Teach

Subject: client

Outcome: pain reduction through use of guided imagery

Target Time: 9/4/91

Signature: Kathy Mayer, RN

•4. Nursing Order

Measurable verb: Discuss

Subject: with client and husband

Outcome: pre/intra/postoperative care mastectomy client

Target time: 9/3/91

Signature: Kathy Mayer, RN

Exercise Q: Writing a Nursing Care Plan for Case Study #1 using *Altered Protection* as the High Priority Nursing Diagnosis,
p. 101-102

ASSESSMENT

Subjective Data

"My knuckles are swollen."

"I have pain, redness, and warmth over my knuckles."

"I had an infected bunion on my left foot."

Objective Data

WBC 11,000

Culture positive staphylococcus

Edema, redness metacarpal phalanges

DYSFUNCTIONAL HEALTH PATTERN

Health Management/Health Perception

NURSING DIAGNOSTIC STATEMENT

Nursing Diagnosis
Altered Protection

Etiology (related to)
immunosuppression

Defining Characteristics (as evidenced by)
increase in WBC, edema, redness joints,
positive culture staphylococcus

OUTCOME CRITERIA

1. Client will demonstrate changing of dressing on left bunion accurately by 9/28/91.

2. Client will verbalize signs and symptoms of infection unassisted by 9/20/91.

3. Client will verbalize the role of protein in tissue regeneration accurately by 9/10/91.

NURSING ORDERS (for)

Outcome Criteria 1:
A: Teach client and wife to change dressing on busion by 9/20/91. Cyndie Smith, RN

Outcome Criteria 2:
B: Teach client and wife early signs of inflammation and infection, by 9/1/0/91. Cyndie Smith, RN

Outcome Criteria 3:
C: Teach the client and wife the basic 4 food groups by 9/12/91. Cyndie Smith, RN

RATIONALE (for)

Nursing Order A:
Medical asepsis limits the number of microorganisms and their spread.

Nursing Order B:
Open wounds are portals of entry for microorganisms. Hand washing is the most effective means of controlling the spread of microorganisms.

Nursing Order C:
A balanced diet supplies essential proteins and vitamins to build new tissue.

Exercise Q: Writing a Nursing Care Plan for Case Study #1 using *Pain* as the High Priority Nursing Diagnosis, p. 101-102

ASSESSMENT

Subjective Data

"It feels like a knife is stabbing each joint."

"I rate my pain an 8."

"This time, the pain was not relieved with ecotrin."

"It hurts when you move my joints."

Objective Data

Facial grimacing.

Moaning when each joint tested for ROM.

Salicylate level 23 mg/dL.

DYSFUNCTIONAL HEALTH PATTERN

Cognitive Perceptual

OUTCOME CRITERIA

1. Client will verbalize pain rating before pain reaches a 4 by 9/3/91.

2. Client will practice slow rhythmic breathing independently by 9/4/91.

3. Client will identify factors that exacerbate the pain realistically by 9/4/91.

NURSING DIAGNOSTIC STATEMENT

Nursing Diagnosis

Pain

Etiology (related to)

chronic disease

Defining Characteristics (as evidenced by)

verbalizations of pain upon joint movement, rated pain intensity an 8, facial grimacing

NURSING ORDERS (for)

Outcome Criteria 1:

A: Teach the client to rate pain intensity on scale of 0-10 by 9/3/91. Cyndie Smith, RN

Outcome Criteria 2:

B: Teach the client slow rhythmic breathing by 9/3/91. Cyndie Smith, RN

Outcome Criteria 3:

C: Evaluate client's pain management by 9/4/91. Cyndie Smith, RN

RATIONALE (for)

Nursing Order A:

The intensity or severity of pain is subjective. The pain rating scale is designed to assist clients in describing the intensity of their pain.

Nursing Order B:

Relaxation techniques are effective in reducing anxiety, muscle tension, and dissociation from the pain.

Nursing Order C:

Establishing a pain management program will lead to realistic pain control goals.

Exercise R: Writing a Nursing Care Plan for Case Study #2 using *Fluid Volume Deficit* as the High Priority Nursing Diagnosis, p. 103-104

ASSESSMENT

Subjective Data

"I drink 2 juice glasses of water a day."

"I do not use diuretics."

"I am thirsty."

Objective Data

Skin turgor: shape returned in 10 seconds.
Hematocrit 50%.
Intake below normal value of 1200cc/qd.

DYSFUNCTIONAL DIAGNOSTIC DIVISION
Food-Fluid

OUTCOME CRITERA

1. Client will demonstrate fluid and electrolyte balance WNL during the perioperative period.

2. Client will verbalize factors leading to fluid volume deficit accurately by 9/4/91.

3. Client will verbalize the amount of fluid necessary to maintain fluid balance by 9/4/91.

NURSING DIAGNOSTIC STATEMENT

Nursing Diagnosis
Fluid Volume Deficit

Etiology (related to)
deviation from normal fluid intake

Defining Characteristics (as evidenced by)
intake below normal 1200 cc/qd, decreased skin turgor, Hct 50%.

NURSING ORDERS (for)
Outcome Criteria 1:
A: Monitor skin turgor, urine specific gravity, Hct, electrolytes, 24 hour intake and output by 9/3/91. Kathy Mayer, RN

Outcome Criteria 2:
B: Evaluate with client factors effecting fluid and electrolyte balance by 9/4/91. Kathy Mayer, RN

Outcome Criteria 3:
C: Teach the client normal fluid intake by 9/4/91. Kathy Mayer, RN

RATIONALE (for)
Nursing Order A:
A balance of fluids and electrolytes is necessary for health and life. The balance of fluids and electrolytes in the body maintains physiologic homeostasis.

Nursing Order B:
Stress affect's a client's fluid and electrolyte balance. The overall response of the body to stress is to increase the blood volume.

Nursing Order C:
The normal daily fluid intake is 2500cc. The source of the intake is fluids, solid food, and water from oxidation. The normal output per day is 2500 cc.

Exercise R: Writing a Nursing Care Plan for Case Study #2 using *Ineffective Airway Clearance* as the High Priority Nursing Diagnosis, p. 103-104

ASSESSMENT

Subjective Data

"I have hay fever."

"I wheeze when I have an asthma attack and get short of breath."

"My eyes and nose have been itching and watering this week."

Objective Data

Respirations 24; minimal wheezing on expiration both lungs; nasal mucosa pale and edematous.

DYSFUNCTIONAL DIAGNOSTIC DIVISION

Ventilation

NURSING DIAGNOSTIC STATEMENT

Nursing Diagnosis

Ineffective Airway Clearance

Etiology (related to)

excess thick secretions

Defining Characteristics (as evidenced by)

nasal mucosa edematous, respirations 24, nasal drainage

OUTCOME CRITERIA

1. Client will deep breath and cough using abdominal muscles 5 min q1h by 9/3/91.

2. Client will demonstrate use of nebulizer accurately by 9/5/91.

3. Client will verbalize effect of medications on breathing pattern by 9/5/91.

NUIRSING ORDERS (for)

Outcome Criteria 1:

A: Teach client therapeutic effects of ventilating lungs today. Kathy Mayer, RN

Outcome Criteria 2:

B: Teach client to slow deep breath with each whiff from nebulizer by 9/3/91. Kathy Mayer, RN

Outcome Criteria 3:

C: Instruct client to hold breath 10 sec when inhaling alupent; wait 2 min between inhalations by 9/3/91. Kathy Mayer, RN

RATIONALE (for)

Nursing Order A:

Deep breathing helps to remove mucous, aerate the lung tissue, and prevent pneumonia.

Nursing Order B:

Deep breath ensures maximum inflation of alveoli.

Nursing Order C:

Increased therapeutic effect of drug is achieved when administered properly.

Exercise R: Writing a Nursing Care Plan for Case Study #2 using *Pain* as the High Priority Nursing Diagnosis, P. 103-104

ASSESSMENT

Subjective Data

"I have hay fever."

"I wheeze when I have an asthma attack and get short of breath."

"My eyes and nose have been itching and watering this week."

Objective Data

Respirations 24; minimal wheezing on expiration both lungs; nasal mucosa pale and edematous.

DYSFUNCTIONAL DIAGNOSTIC DIVISION

Pain

NURSING DIAGNOSTIC STATEMENT

Nursing Diagnosis
Pain

Etiology (related to)
physiological injuring agent

Defining Characteristics (as evidenced by)
rated pain 7, facial grimacing, palpable neck and shoulder muscles

OUTCOME CRITERIA

1. Client will verbalize pain rating before pain reaches a 4 by 9/4/91.

2. Client will practice guided imagery and rhythmic breathing at onset of migraine by 9/4/91.

3. Client will verbalize factors that trigger her migraine headaches by 9/4/91.

NUIRSING ORDERS (for)

Outcome Criteria 1:
A: Teach client to rate pain on scale 0-10 by 9/3/91. Kathy Mayer, RN

Outcome Criteria 2:
B: Teach the client pain reduction through the use of guided imagery and rhythmic breathing by 9/4/91. Kathy Mayer, RN

Outcome Criteria 3:
C:Evaluate client's pain management plan by 9/3/91. Kathy Mayer, RN

RATIONALE (for)

Nursing Order A:
The intensity or severity of pain is subjective. The pain rating scale is designed to assist the clients in describing the intensity of their pain.

Nursing Order B:
Relaxation techniques are effective in reducing stress, anxiety, muscle tension, and dissociation from the pain.

Nursing Order C:
Identifying stress factors that trigger the migraine headaches, will lead to the establishment of a realistic pain management program.

Exercise S: Independent Nursing Actions p. 107

1. Teach the client and wife to change dressing on bunion

2. Teach client pain reduction through rhythmic breathing wrist/foot; 9/1/91 WBC 11,000; culture positive staph.

3. Demonstrate medical aseptic technique in cleansing mouth

4. Demonstrate safe ambulating techniques with a walker

Exercise T: Independent Nursing Actions p. 108

1. Teach client relaxation techniques.

2. Explain and demonstrate therapeutic effects deep breathing/coughing q1h.

3. Monitor intake and output; blood chemistry/hematology values fall within normal values.

4. Teach client pain reduction through use guided imagery

Exercise U: Narrative Nurses Notes p. 117

Date	Time	
9/4/91	1230	Nurses note: Pain
		Stated, "I am having pain in all my joints. I rate my pain an 8 on scale 0-
		10. I take ecotrin 20-24 tablets day at home. I need some Tylenol #3 for
		this pain. It feels like a knife s stabbing each joint." Moaning, facial
		muscles taut. BP 160/80, P 100, R 22. Cyndie Smith, RN
9/4/91	1245	Nurses note: Pain
		Tylenol #3 Tab. 2 (o) given. Cyndie Smith, RN
9/4/91	1315	Nurses note: Pain
		Stated, "I feel better. I rate my pain a 4 on scale 0-10." BP 140/80, P 80, R 18.
		No facial grimacing. Taught distraction techniques to alleviate pain.
		Cyndie Smith, RN

Exercise V: FOCUS Nurses Notes p. 119

Date	Time	
9/4/91	1230	FOCUS: Nurses note: Pain
		DATA: Stated,"I am having pain in all my joints. I rate my pain an 8 on scale 0-10. I take
		ecotrin 20-24 tablets a day at home. I need some tylenol #3 for this pain. It feels like a knife
		is stabbing each joint. Moaning. Facial muscles taut. BP 160/80. P 100. R 22.
		Cyndie Smith, RN
9/4/91	1245	Nurses note: Pain
		ACTION: Tylenol #3 Tabs 2 (o) given. Cyndie Smith, RN
9/4/91	1215	Nurses note: Pain
		RESPONSE: Stated,"I feel better, I rate my pain a 4." No facial grimacing or moaning.
		BP 140/80. P 80. R 18.
		TEACHING: Taught distraction techniques for alleviation of pain. Cyndie Smith, RN

Exercise W: SOAP Nurses Notes p. 121

Date	Time	
9/3/91	1400	Nurses note: Pain

S: "I am having a migraine headache. I feel nauseated. Please give me some medicine. I rate my pain a 7. It feels like pressure over my left eye and causes my eye to tear. I am so tense about this surgery. Aspirin does not help. I take ergotamine one tablet when my headache begins. "

O: Diaphoretic. Facial grimacing. Tearing left eye. Rubbing left forehead. Palpable neck and shoulder muscles. Lights off in room shades on window pulled. BP 146/80 lying. P 90. R 20.

A: No relief from migraine. Pain persists.

P: Administer pain medication. Teach distraction techniques. Kathy Mayer, RN

9/4/91	1415	Nurses note: Pain

Ergotamine 2mg sublingual administered. Kathy Mayer, RN

9/4/91	1500	Nurses note: Pain

S: "My migraine is a little better. I rate the pain a 4. My nausea is gone."

O: No facial grimacing. No diaphoresis. No rubbing left forehead.

A: Relief obtained from pain medication.

P: Teach use guided imagery to alleviate pain. Kathy Mayer, RN

Exercise X: Evaluating the Achievement of Outcome Criteria p. 127

1. Outcome Criterion: Client and wife will demonstrate changing of dressing on bunion accurately by 9/20/91.

Resolved: YES X   NO __

Evaluation: Wife demonstrated changing of sterile dressing on bunion accurately. Client unable to perform task due to limited joint mobility.

2. Outcome Criterion: Client will practice slow rhythmic breathing independently before pain rating reaches 4 by 9/4/91.

Resolved: YES X_   NO __

Evaluation: Client observed practicing slow rhythmic breathing independently an average of 4 times during the am and pm shifts; and utilized during the night as sleep aid. Client verbalized, "For the majority of the time, I keep my pain rating to a 3 using the rhythmic breathing."

3. Outcome Criterion: Client will rinse buccal mucosa, tongue, and gums with saline after each meal and at bedtime by 9/5/91.

Resolved: YES X_   NO __

Evaluation: Client observed rinsing mouth with saline after each meal and at bedtime. Due to limited joint mobility, client expressed verbal difficulty in handling the glass. Upon observation, client was able to put glass to mouth, rinse mouth, and expectorate saline without assistance. Buccal lesions persist. Rinses will be continued.

4. Outcome Criterion: Client will walk with a walker unassisted 20 feet, 4 times a day by 9/14/91.

Resolved: YES X_   NO __

Evaluation: By 9/14/91, client demonstrated the ability to walk with a walker unassisted, 20 feet, 4-6 times a day. Client verbalized a feeling of increased strength in quadricep muscles.

Exercise Y: Evaluation the Achievement of Outcome Criteria p. 129

1. Outcome Criterion: Explain and demonstrate to client the therapeutic effects of deep breathing/coughing q1h

9/3/91

Resolved: YES X   NO X

Evaluation: Client observed deep breathing and coughing q1h postoperatively. Lungs clear to auscultation. No edema nasal turbinates. No nasal drainage. R 18.

2. Outcome Criterion: Monitor client's intake and output; blood chemistry/hematology values fall within normal

values.

Resolved: YES X   NO __

Evaluation: Fluid and electrolytes, and hematology values within normal limits by surgery 9/5/91, and within normal limits at discharge.

3. Outcome Criterion: Client will practice guided imagery at onset migraine and q1h until migraine pain is rated

below a 4.

Resolved: YES __   NO X

Evaluation: Client practiced guided imagery sporadically during the postoperative period. Husband not present during the preoperative and intraoperative periods. Husband present postoperatively. Husband and wife taught imagery.

4. Outcome Criterion: Client and husband will describe postoperative outcomes, possible complications, and

discharge planning realistically and accurately before scheduled surgery.

Resolved: YES __   NO X

Evaluation: Surgeon discussed postoperative outcomes and possible complications with client. Husband not present pre/intraoperatively. Discharge planning discussed with client and husband postoperatively. Client demonstrates unrealistic expectations of self and plans to return to work in 2 weeks.

Bibliography

Allen, C.V. (1988) *Nursing Process Workbook.* Detroit: Allen.

Allen, C.V. (1990). The Art of Observation. *Nursing Times,* 86(2), 36-37.

Allen, C.V. (1990). Art in Nursing. *American Journal of Nursing,* 90(2), 34.

American Nurses' Association. (1973). *Standards of Nursing Practice.* Missouri: American Nurses' Association

American Nurses' Association. (1980). *The American Nurses' Association Social Policy Statement.* Missouri: American Nurses' Association.

Black, H., Nolan, J., & Nolan-Haley, J. (1990). *Black's Law Dictionary* (6th ed.). Minnesota: West.

Doenges, M., & Moorhouse, M. (1989). *Psychiatric Care Plans: Guidelines for Patient Care.* Philadelphia: Davis.

Doenges, M. & Moorhouse, M. (1988). *Nurse's Pocket Guide: Nursing Diagnoses with Interventions* (2nd Ed.). Philadelphia: Davis.

Goodman, L.S., & Gillman, A. (1990). *The Pharmacological Basis of Therapeutics* (8th ed.). New York: Pergamon.

Gordon, M. (1989). *Manual of Nursing Diagnosis 1988-1989.* St. Louis: Mosby-Year Book, Inc.

Gordon, M. (1987). *Nursing Diagnosis: Process and Application* (2nd ed.). St. Louis: Mosby-Year Book, Inc.

Joint Commission of Accreditation of Healthcare Organizations (1991). *1991 Accreditation Manual for Hospitals.* Chicago: Joint Commission of Accreditation of Healthcare Organizations.

Kee, J.L. (1990). *Handbook of Laboratory and Diagnostic Tests with Nursing Implications.* Connecticut: Appleton & Lange.

Kozier, B., & Erb, G. (1987). *Fundamentals of Nursing* (2nd ed.). California: Addison-Wesley.

Lewis, S., & Collier, I. (1987). *Medical-Surgical Nursing Assessment and Management of Clinical Problems* (2nd ed.). St. Louis: Mosby-Year Book, Inc.

Miller, M., & Malcolm, N. (1990). Critical Thinking in the Nursing Curriculum. *Nursing & Health Care,* 11(2), 67-73.

North American Nurses Diagnosis Association. (1990). *Taxonomy I-Revised 1990.* St. Louis: North American Nurses Diagnosis Association.

Sherman, J.L., & Fields, S.K. (1988). *Guide to Patient Evaluation: History Taking a Physical Examination and the Nursing Process* (5th ed.). New York: Medical Examination.

Index